Dr. Anderson's
HIGH-FIBER
FITNESS
PLAN

Dr. Anderson's

HIGH - FIBER FITNESS PLAN

James W. Anderson, M.D.

with Nancy J. Gustafson, M.S., R.D.

THE UNIVERSITY PRESS OF KENTUCKY

Scholarly publisher for the Commonwealth,
serving Bellarmine College, Berea College, Centre
College of Kentucky, Eastern Kentucky University,
The Filson Club, Georgetown College, Kentucky
Historical Society, Kentucky State University,
Morehead State University, Murray State University,
Northern Kentucky University, Transylvania University,
University of Kentucky, University of Louisville,
and Western Kentucky University.

Editorial and Sales Offices: Lexington, Kentucky 40508-4008

Library of Congress Cataloging-in-Publication Data

Anderson, James W.
    [High-fiber fitness plan]
    Dr. Anderson's high-fiber fitness plan / James W. Anderson with
Nancy J. Gustafson.
        p.   cm.
    Includes index.
    ISBN 0-8131-1867-0 (acid-free paper)
    1. High-fiber diet—Recipes.   I. Gustafson, Nancy J.   II. Title.
III. Title: Doctor Anderson's high-fiber fitness plan.
RM237.6.A53   1994
613.2'6—dc20   93–45451

To Gay, Kathy, and Steve

Contents

Preface

ARE YOU AT RISK for having a heart attack? Has someone in your family had cancer? Do you have a friend with diabetes? Chances are that the answers to these questions are yes. All of us have a high risk for heart attack and cancer and a moderate risk for diabetes since these commonly occur in American adults. Fortunately, these diseases can be controlled and even prevented with good diet and lifestyle habits.

If you are a busy person who likes good food but doesn't like to spend much time preparing it, this book is for you. If you are healthy now, this book will give you fresh and simple ideas on good eating and living to stay well. If you have a few extra pounds to lose, you'll appreciate the book's positive, nonrestrictive approach. If you are developing some health problems, this book is especially for you.

Our Metabolic Research Team at the University of Kentucky has studied ways to prevent and treat chronic diseases for twenty years. In 1973, we started testing foods high in carbohydrate and fiber to treat people with diabetes. Not only did a high-fiber diet improve blood sugar levels in these individuals, but, much to our surprise, their blood cholesterol levels went down also.

Then I became the first human guinea pig to try oat bran, which I guessed would lower my own high cholesterol level inherited from my mother. In 1977, I contacted the Quaker Oats Company about the possibility of getting oat bran for research purposes.

Today you can buy oat bran in any grocery store, but in 1977 even Quaker Oats in Chicago had not heard of it. After two calls and some checking, the Quaker people referred me to their milling plant in Cedar Rapids, Iowa. The miller told me that oat bran was a by-product of making oat flour for face powder; he agreed to send me one hundred pounds of it.

In the interest of science, I began eating a large bowl of oat bran each morning and three to four oat bran muffins each day. During the five-week test period, my cholesterol dropped from 285 to 175 milligrams per deciliter and I lost eight pounds without greatly changing my other eating habits.

Compelled by my own experience, we began testing the cholesterol-lowering effects of oat bran for real people—those with diabetes and then for people with high cholesterol levels. These studies set the stage for the enormous popularity of oat bran in the 1980s.

Since these early days with oat bran we have experimented with new types of fibers such as those in grains, beans, fruits, and vegetables. We have also studied high-fiber plant extracts such as psyllium and guar gum. The studies of our Metabolic Research Team are recognized worldwide, and the National Institute of Health has supported our fiber research with over $1.5 million in grant money.

Our research and recommendations have evolved over the years to include a healthy variety of food fibers and their effects on several chronic diseases. We have developed and refined a high-fiber disease prevention plan that is delicious, simple, and practical, yet highly effective. I have seen hundreds of individuals on this plan lose weight without trying, drop their cholesterol level 50 points or more, cut their risk for heart disease in half, normalize their blood pressure, control their blood sugar, reduce their cancer risk, stop medications, and start enjoying life more.

Now for the first time ever we have simplified our prevention plan and tailored it to busy working people. Many books tell you what *not* to eat. In this book we'll tell you what *to* eat, and no foods are off limits. All the recipes in this book contain less than 30 percent of calories as fat, so you can eat as much as you want without worrying much about the calories.

Experts across the country and abroad support the recommendations made in this book. The American Heart, Dietetic, and Diabetes associations, the National Cancer Institute, the U.S. Department of Agriculture, and health experts in Great Britain and Canada all arrived at the same conclusion: the healthiest kind of diet that fights chronic disease is high in carbohydrate and fiber and low in fat.

As a person who knows what it's like to struggle with weight and high blood cholesterol, and as a doctor who has helped thousands of individuals dramatically improve their health, I am convinced that a sensible eating and lifestyle plan such as the one in this book will substantially improve your health and will be easier than you think.

Note: The information in this book should not replace regular medical care. Please consult your own doctor as you begin our prevention plan.

HEALTH-PROMOTING FOODS AND PRACTICES

1
FIBER FIGHTS
THE FAMOUS FIVE

SUCCESS STORY:
Bill reverses diabetes and high blood fats.

Bill* was only forty-one years old and just thirty-three pounds overweight when he came to see me as a patient. The week before he literally had run to my office after receiving results of routine blood tests ordered by his regular doctor. His blood values after twelve hours without food were: cholesterol, 278 mg/dl (milligrams per deciliter); triglycerides, 645 mg/dl; and glucose, 288 mg/dl. All these values were abnormally high, meaning Bill not only was flirting with a heart attack but also had diabetes.

Bill considered himself to be very healthy and had no past medical problems. His blood test results seemed especially unexpected considering he was a highly successful cardiologist who worked in the same medical center as I did.

Bill ran the coronary care unit and the helicopter transport service at our medical center. He was the only senior doctor who regularly flew in the helicopter to pick up heart-attack victims in remote areas of Eastern Kentucky—a high-stress position. Bill also conducted excellent clinical research into new types of heart catheters and was in high demand to share this new technology.

We made an appointment and I saw Bill in my office the next week. We went over all of his health habits, including the foods he usually ate. His meals were nothing out of the ordinary—ordinary for the typical fat-eating American. He traveled frequently and often ate on airplanes, at medical meetings, and in hotels and restaurants. Except for rushing from hospital to hospital and from airplane to airplane, Bill obtained no regular exercise.

---

* The names used throughout this book have been changed to protect the privacy of individuals and their families.

But while Bill's blood tests had been normal about two years ago, they failed to show the silent changes taking place inside his body. His all-American diet combined with his inactive, stressful lifestyle gradually were narrowing his blood vessels and raising his weight, blood pressure, and blood cholesterol levels. His body also lost the ability to handle carbohydrates (sugars and starches) properly, driving up his blood sugar.

If I had used the typical approach with Bill, I would have put him on a low-fat, low-cholesterol plan such as the American Heart Association diet, and restricted sugar for both his cholesterol and his blood sugar problem. But, as Bill and I both knew, such an approach often brings down cholesterol levels only slightly—5 to 7 percent, according to many well-known studies. And blood sugar often fails to respond to such a diet.

Bill came to me because he knew that our Metabolic Research Team at the University of Kentucky has experienced dramatic success with using unique high-fiber diets to control high cholesterol, diabetes, and other metabolic problems. Many of his patients had responded dramatically to our treatment program. Bill also had read several of our research publications and knew our approach lowered blood cholesterol and glucose levels much more effectively than ordinary approaches.

Bill and I both concluded that his diet and lifestyle had sabotaged his health. Yes, his high fat intake, particularly animal fat, claimed some of the blame. But Bill also needed more fiber, especially a particular type of fiber called soluble fiber. Soluble fiber helps take extra cholesterol out of the body and keeps the body from producing so much cholesterol. Soluble fiber also helps stabilize blood sugar and promotes weight loss and maintenance.

For many of us, knowing the theory behind healthful eating and actually eating that way are quite different. Bill needed help translating our eating recommendations into everyday foods. Bill is a compulsive sort of guy and asked for copies of all our written materials on diet and health. With the help of our registered dietitians, we developed an individualized prevention plan for Bill suited to his habits, food preferences, and lifestyle.

Bill stuck to our prevention plan zealously, even overdoing it at times. In two weeks he came back to see me and we repeated his blood tests, which showed good improvement. In another three weeks we repeated them again. The results even surprised me: Bill's blood cholesterol had dropped to 157 mg/dl, his blood triglycerides to 103 mg/dl, and his blood sugar to 114 mg/dl. All these values were perfectly within the healthy range, and Bill didn't take a single pill to get them there.

At the writing of this book, Bill continues to follow our prevention plan and maintains his weight at about 158 pounds, down from his high of 198 pounds. His blood sugar is a normal 87 mg/dl, his cholesterol is 133 mg/dl—down 145 points— and his triglycerides are 93 mg/dl—down more than 550 points. His low-density lipoprotein levels, the kind of cholesterol that is especially prone to clogging blood vessels, measures unusually low at 76 mg/dl. Bill does not take any medicine and maintains these excellent numbers by following our high-fiber diet and exercising regularly.

BILL'S SCORECARD				
Measurement	**Initial**	**5 weeks on plan**	**1 year on plan**	**Ideal**
Weight, lbs.	198	179	158	165
Glucose, mg/dl	288	114	87	<115
Cholesterol, mg/dl	278	157	133	<200
Triglycerides, mg/dl	645	103	93	<150
Exercise, miles/week	5	33	40	12 to 20

The Famous Five

Diet contributes to the development of five deadly problems: heart disease, cancer, high blood pressure, obesity, and diabetes. The American diet has changed drastically over the last ninety years. Consumption of meat has almost doubled since 1909, and consumption of dairy products has increased 25 percent. Americans eat 50 percent more fats and oils than they did in 1909, with most of the increase coming from margarine and cooking and salad oils.

Although Americans now eat more citrus foods than they used to, consumption of fresh fruits has decreased by 36 percent and consumption of fresh vegetables has decreased by 23 percent. Americans eat 38 percent fewer white potatoes and 79 percent fewer sweet potatoes than they did in 1909. Consumption of grain products has also decreased by about one-half. All these changes translate into more fat and less carbohydrate and fiber in our diet.

During the same ninety years, U.S. rates of chronic diseases have also changed drastically. Since the early 1900s the leading killer diseases gradually shifted from infectious to chronic diseases. U.S. death rates from cancer have more than tripled and death rates from heart disease more than doubled during the same period. The 40 percent drop in deaths from coronary heart disease since the mid-1960s may be partly because of improved medical care and perhaps partly because of better diet habits.

Today five of the ten leading causes of death in the United States are diet related. Heart disease, cancer, stroke (often related to high blood pressure), diabetes (often related to obesity), and atherosclerosis (hardening of the arteries) account for 68 percent of all deaths in the United States. (Of the other five leading causes of death, alcohol use has been found to be a factor in three causes—unintentional injuries, suicide, and liver disease.)

In addition to the five diet-related killers, diet contributes to other diseases that fuel these killers. One in four Americans has high blood pressure, which greatly increases risk of both heart disease and stroke. One in three Americans weighs more than he or she should. Obesity increases risk for all five killer diseases.

An Unprecedented Consensus

Health experts across the country today are rallying efforts to attack and prevent diet-related diseases. In the last decade a broad spectrum of U.S. health organizations reached an unprecedented consensus on healthful eating for chronic disease prevention.

First a U.S. Senate Select Committee developed dietary guidelines for Americans, which advocated increasing intake of complex carbohydrates, naturally occurring sugars, and fiber and limiting fat intake to 30 percent of calories. These guidelines were recently affirmed and updated by the U.S. departments of Agriculture and Health and Human Services.

Next followed a series of diet recommendations for prevention or treatment of specific diseases. The National Cancer Institute recommended a fiber intake of 20 to 30 grams daily and advocated eating fiber from a variety of food sources, including vegetables, fruits, and whole-grain cereals.

The American Diabetes Association recommended eating 40 grams of fiber daily, getting 55 to 60 percent of calories from carbohydrate, and substituting unrefined carbohydrates, which contain fiber for low-fiber, highly refined carbohydrates. The American Heart Association made no specific recommendations for fiber intake but recommended a diet high in complex carbohydrates and low in fat and cholesterol. More recently, a report of the surgeon general recommended that Americans increase their intake of whole-grain foods and cereal products, vegetables (including dried beans and peas), and fruits.

It's no coincidence that all these recommendations sound alike. Scientists have reached an unprecedented consensus: the best type of diet to prevent chronic diseases is low in fat and includes generous amounts of plant foods, which are high in fiber.

Focus on Fiber

For millennia, the benefits of healthful eating have been widely recognized. In the Old Testament, Daniel insisted on eating his traditional diet of pulses (legumes such as beans, lentils, and peas) and water instead of the rich food of the king of Babylon. After ten days on the legumes and water, Daniel and his friends looked healthier than the young men who were eating the king's rich food. This is one of the earliest experiments showing the benefits of a high-fiber diet.

However, fiber got very little respect until the 1970s when evidence began to emerge documenting its nutritional value. Prior to that time, fiber was thought of as just the roughage in plant foods, which the body could not fully digest.

Then in the mid 1970s two British physicians reported exceptionally low rates of chronic killer diseases among Africans who ate large amounts of high-fiber foods. About this same time, a few researchers in the United States, including our team, and Great Britian started exploring the use of fiber in treating diseases. Since these early pioneering studies hundreds of other studies have confirmed the role of high-fiber foods in disease prevention and treatment.

Two main types of fiber are found in plant foods—soluble and insoluble. Animal foods, of course, contain no plant fiber. Soluble fibers are gummy, gelling-type fibers found more in fruits, some vegetables, dried beans and peas, and oat products. Insoluble fibers account for about 70 percent of the fiber in our diets, are present in all plant foods, and are concentrated in wheat bran. Both types of fiber play important roles in disease prevention.

Fiber and Heart Disease

Despite a drop in death rates from heart disease in recent years, heart disease still remains the number one killer in America. It claims more than five hundred thousand lives and costs more than $110 billion yearly in health care expenses and lost productivity.

Several factors influence heart disease, including genetic and environmental factors. Older people, men, and black individuals are more susceptible to heart disease. Although the risk of heart disease is lower in middle-aged women than men, risk rises after menopause, and heart disease is still the leading killer in women. For comparison, heart disease kills six times more American women than does breast cancer; cardiovascular disease, including heart attack and stroke, kills four times more American women than do breast and lung cancer combined.

Of the environmental factors we can control, the three major risk factors for heart disease are high blood cholesterol levels, high blood pressure, and cigarette smoking. Each of these risk factors more than triples the risk for heart attack or stroke. If someone has all three of these risk factors, the chances of experiencing a heart attack or stroke increase fifteenfold.

High blood cholesterol levels can clog blood vessels, contributing to hardening of the arteries or atherosclerosis. Eventually cholesterol and other fatty deposits can totally block blood flow or break loose and become lodged in another blood vessel. If blood flow to a portion of the heart stops, a heart attack occurs. If blood flow to part of the brain stops, a stroke occurs. Obesity, inactivity, and high blood glucose (diabetes) also contribute to heart disease, both independently and through their effects on blood cholesterol and blood pressure levels.

The American Heart Association recommends a low-fat, low-cholesterol diet for individuals with or at risk of heart disease. Such diets, however, have been shown to lower blood cholesterol levels only 5 to 7 percent. Emphasizing foods high in fiber, particularly soluble fiber, lowers cholesterol levels even farther than an American Heart Association-type diet. In our studies, low-fat, low-cholesterol diets that include up to 50 grams of fiber daily lower blood cholesterol levels 20 to 30 percent. Since every 1 percent drop in blood cholesterol results in a 2 percent drop in risk for heart disease, this translates into an estimated 40 to 60 percent reduction in heart disease risk for our patients who maintain the high-fiber prevention program.

In one of our typical studies of men with high cholesterol levels, increasing fiber by using one serving of either oat bran or dried beans daily lowered blood cholesterol 19 percent in three weeks and maintained even greater reductions over the long term. Blood levels of low-density lipoprotein, a particular type of blood cholesterol especially prone to clogging blood vessels, also fell quickly and remained 24 percent lower after twenty-four weeks on the diet and 29 percent lower after ninety-nine weeks on the diet.

We like to see our patients lower their cholesterol levels to below 200 mg/dl, since risk for heart disease sharply rises with cholesterol levels above 200 mg/dl. Most of our patients respond nicely to our prevention combination of diet and lifestyle habits.

When he began his prevention plan, Bill's cholesterol dropped from 278 to 157 mg/dl, lowering his cholesterol 43 percent. If he can sustain these levels, his risk for heart disease could be reduced as much as 80 percent. When I first began eating oat bran regularly in 1977, my cholesterol fell from 285 to 175 mg/dl—a 39 percent drop that should reduce my heart disease risk by up to 78 percent.

Studies have also suggested that fiber may reduce risk for heart disease independent of its effects on blood cholesterol. In two separate studies, one in England and one in the Netherlands, men with the lowest cereal fiber intake had five times the rate of heart disease that men with the highest cereal fiber intake had. In a study of twenty developed countries, countries with the lowest fiber intakes from vegetables, fruits, grains, and legumes had the highest death rates from heart disease. In this study, the United States ranked lowest in fiber intake and highest in heart disease death rate.

Fiber and High Blood Pressure

High blood pressure, or hypertension, is a major risk factor for both heart disease and stroke. One in four white Americans and one in three black Americans suffers from high blood pressure. The incidence rises with age.

With high blood pressure, the heart must pump harder than normal to circulate blood through the body. This strains the heart and wears and tears the blood vessels, contributing to hardening of the arteries, heart attack, and stroke.

Vegetarians with high fiber intakes have lower blood pressure levels than nonvegetarians of the same sex and age with low fiber intakes. In our studies, high-fiber diets lower blood pressures of people in both groups by about 10 percent: the systolic or upper numbers decrease 12 to 15 points (millimeters of mercury or mm Hg) while the diastolic or lower numbers decrease 7 to 9 points. In our experience, even modest increases in fiber intake result in distinct falls in blood pressure.

Several other researchers have reported that high-fiber diets lower blood pressure, but the independent effects of fiber are hard to sort out from other aspects of a high-fiber diet. The low fat and sodium content and the high potassium, magnesium, and calcium content of vegetarian diets may contribute to lower blood pressure. Regardless of the cause, however, diets generous in plant foods and fiber decrease systolic blood pressure by 6 to 10 points and diastolic blood pressure by 4 to 6 points.

Fiber and Cancer

Cancer is a close second to heart disease in the number of American lives it claims each year. Costs for cancer exceed $70 billion yearly counting direct health care expenses and lost productivity. Up to 70 percent of all cancer deaths each year could have been prevented with better diet and lifestyle habits.

The National Cancer Institute's dietary guidelines advocate a fiber intake of 20 to 30 grams daily. In a Dutch study, men with low fiber intakes had three times the death rate from cancer compared to men with high fiber intakes.

Fiber may protect against certain cancers in several ways. Fiber has been suggested to protect against colon cancer, perhaps by diluting cancer-causing agents in the colon. One study noted that Danish individuals with low fiber intakes developed colon cancer three times more frequently than Finnish individuals with high fiber intakes. Other studies associate breast cancer with high fat and low fiber intake.

Vitamins C and E and beta carotene, a compound that can be converted into vitamin A in the body, may also help prevent certain cancers. A high intake of these vitamins is associated with low rates of several types of cancers. These vitamins act as antioxidants, which may protect body cells from injuries that can give rise to cancer. The oxygen we breathe is vital to many body functions, but oxygen can be converted into highly toxic chemicals called free radicals. Various antioxidants in the body protect us from damage from these toxic free radicals. Vegetables, fruits, and whole grains are important sources of beta carotene as well as vitamins C and E, which are potent antioxidants.

Most fiber-rich foods such as fruits and vegetables are also rich in antioxidants. In fact, the National Cancer Institute recently introduced a multimillion dollar national campaign to get Americans to eat more fruits and vegetables. The campaign, called "Five a Day for Better Health," advocates eating a minimum of five servings of fruits and vegetables daily to help prevent cancer.

Fiber and Obesity

Obesity affects thirty-four million American adults and an increasing number of American children. The number of Americans who weigh more than they should is growing. Americans spend billions of dollars each year on diet programs and products in search of thinness. Of those who lose significant weight, only 5 percent maintain their weight loss long term. Losing weight is not the cure; weight loss must be maintained.

Obesity raises risk of most other chronic diseases, including heart disease, high blood pressure, diabetes, and perhaps breast and colon cancer. Death rates of individuals who weigh 50 percent more than they should (for most of us, that's sixty to ninety pounds) are twice that of individuals at their ideal body weight. Up to age seventy, losing even 10 percent of body weight, or fifteen to twenty pounds, can significantly improve life expectancy. After age seventy we do not recommend a weight-reduction program unless you are more than fifty pounds overweight or have serious medical problems necessitating weight loss.

High-fiber foods are usually low in fat and calories and promote weight loss. They take longer to eat, they slow the emptying of the stomach, and they lower blood levels of insulin, an appetite-stimulating hormone. Nutrients such as starch may also be less well absorbed into the body from high-fiber foods, providing slightly fewer calories than comparable low-fiber foods.

In our studies with overweight men, 2,000-calorie diets high in fiber produced weight losses of about two pounds per week, while 1,200-calorie high-fiber diets produced weight losses of about four pounds per week. We also used severely restricted 800-calorie high-fiber diets, which produced weight losses of six to seven pounds per week, but we don't recommend dropping your calories this low without careful medical supervision.

Fiber and Diabetes

Diabetes is a disease in which the body cannot handle sugar properly, either because of a total lack or insufficiency of a hormone called insulin or because the body becomes resistant to insulin's action. Insulin is one of the main hormones that regulate blood sugar, acting as a key to let sugar into the cells to be burned for energy. Without proper amounts or proper functioning of insulin, blood sugar rises to dangerously high levels because it cannot get into the cells.

Health professionals recognize two distinct types of diabetes. In the first type, insulin-dependent or type I diabetes, the body totally loses its ability to make insulin. In the second type, non–insulin-dependent or type II diabetes, the body does not make enough insulin or becomes resistant to insulin's action. Type I diabetes usually comes on suddenly in childhood or early adulthood, while type II diabetes can develop more gradually and later in life.

Of the approximately fourteen million Americans with diabetes, including one-third who don't even know they have the disease, 90 percent have type II diabetes. Of these 90 percent, most are overweight. In fact, reducing to a more desirable body weight is the main treatment of individuals with type II diabetes.

Getting sugar to all those extra fat cells becomes more than the body's usual supply of insulin can handle in overweight individuals with type II diabetes. To make things worse, in obesity, the body cells become resistant to insulin's action. Often when a person with type II diabetes loses weight, the insulin resistance improves and the available insulin once again becomes adequate, reversing the disease. With intensive diet intervention we stop insulin treatment in two-thirds of the type II diabetic individuals that we treat.

Diabetes also accelerates hardening of the arteries and is a risk factor for heart disease. Diabetic men are twice as likely and diabetic women are four times as likely to have a heart attack as are nondiabetic men and women. Individuals with diabetes often have high blood fat levels, tend to have high blood pressure, and are usually more overweight than nondiabetic individuals.

High-fiber diets improve diabetic control in three ways and may even produce a complete remission in type II diabetes. First, high-fiber diets, especially those rich in soluble fiber, lower blood fat levels, reducing risk for heart disease. Second, high-fiber diets promote weight loss and maintenance, lessening insulin insufficiency and resistance. Finally, fiber acts independently to lower blood sugar and improve the action of insulin.

In our studies, high-fiber diets lowered insulin requirements of individuals with type I diabetes an average of 38 percent. For individuals with type II diabetes, such diets lowered insulin requirements an average of 97 percent, meaning most type II diabetic individuals using insulin or diabetes pills were able to stop these treatments and still maintain a healthy blood sugar level. Individuals in our study have continued to maintain good diabetic control on these lowered or discontinued insulin doses for up to fifteen years as long as they continue the high-fiber diet. Recent studies from other centers suggest that high-fiber diets reduce risk for eye disease and kidney damage in diabetics.

Fiber and hypoglycemia

SUCCESS STORY:
Marcie corrects low blood sugar.

Marcie, a nineteen-year-old college student, came to see me because of fainting spells. For six years she had suffered from weak spells, episodes of shakiness, and occasional fainting. These episodes came on between meals and could be prevented by drinking fruit juice or eating crackers. Marcie had undergone extensive medical testing, including evaluation for a brain tumor. Previously she had been instructed to eat a high-protein diet, which had increased the frequency and intensity of her spells.

Her physical examination was normal, but laboratory studies confirmed the diagnosis of reactive hypoglycemia, meaning low blood sugar occuring between meals. Her low blood sugar was due to the sluggish release of insulin from the pancreas. After a meal her body released insulin later than normal, causing her blood sugar to drop to an abnormally low level before the next meal.

The dietitian instructed Marcie on our high-fiber diet program tailored to the low blood sugar problem and encouraged her to exercise regularly. Marcie's frequency of weak spells decreased immediately, and after three weeks she stopped having weak spells and episodes of shakiness. Over the next eighteen months she had no more fainting spells and only occasional weak spells. Marcie joins the list of dozens of young people and adults who have stabilized their blood sugar through our prevention diet and exercise plan. High fiber intake slows the emptying of the stomach, delays absorption of sugar into body cells, and minimizes blood sugar swings. In our experience, almost all individuals with hypoglycemia respond favorably to our prevention plan.

Fiber and Other Diseases

When British researchers first proposed a link between high fiber intake and low rates of chronic disease, they also noted the low incidence of hiatal hernia, appendicitis, diverticular disease of the colon, constipation, irritable colon, bowel polyps, and hemorrhoids among populations with high fiber intake. While the link between fiber and most of these diseases remains to be proven, fiber does play a well-documented role in treating constipation.

Constipation can be a major problem for some people and contributes to hemorrhoids, varicose veins, and diverticular disease of the colon. High fiber intake, particularily from wheat bran or psyllium, increases stool bulk and speeds up stool passage through the intestines.

How to Use This Book

Improving your health and helping you get the most out of life is the goal of this book. If you are healthy now, we want you to stay that way. If you are overweight or have heart disease, high blood pressure, low blood sugar, or diabetes, following our high-fiber prevention plan can improve your symptoms and may even reverse your disease.

You are busy, we know, and don't have extra time to spend shopping, planning menus, and cooking meals. Few people cook gourmet today except for occasional social events. Our prevention plan is designed for people who like good food and like to eat but have little time to spend preparing food. It emphasizes what to eat instead of what not to eat and directs you to health-promoting foods and practices.

We'll get right to the heart of our plan in the next chapter. The prevention plan is a simple, nonrestrictive, and satisfying plan that combines good eating with regular exercise and healthful lifestyle habits.

If you are anxious to lose weight fast or need to get problems from heart disease, high blood pressure, or diabetes under control quickly, we recommend following our slightly more structured quick loss plan in chapter 3. You can follow the quick loss plan until you lose the weight you want to, then switch to the lifetime prevention plan.

To save you time and energy, we've simplified shopping, cooking, and eating out. Chapter 5 gives you an aisle-by-aisle grocery guide emphasizing convenient yet healthful choices for busy lifestyles. We'll also tell you how to get the most out of labels at a glance.

Chapter 6 gives time-saving suggestions for menu planning and food preparation the high-fiber way. Chapter 7 suggests healthful prevention choices for vending machines, cafeterias, traveling, fast food restaurants, and all major restaurant categories.

You will find a week's worth of daily menus of quick and tasty meals that fit our prevention and quick loss plans. Finally, the last section of the book contains over 150 tested and easy-to-make high-fiber recipes, complete with nutritional breakdowns. You won't need your calculator since all our recipes provide less than 30 percent of calories from fat.

We hope we have convinced you of fiber's powerful role in preventing and treating killer diseases. Now let us convince you that our prevention plan is delicious, satisfying, and easy—a way of living we hope you'll get hooked on for life.

2
YOUR LIFETIME DIET PLAN

SUCCESS STORY:
Mary lowers her blood cholesterol.

Mary was thirty-seven years old when she first came to see me five years ago about her high blood cholesterol problem. She was slender, physically active, and healthy, but she was concerned about her blood cholesterol because of her father's heart attack at age sixty-one. Her blood cholesterol was 257 mg/dl, and her LDL cholesterol (the "bad guy") was 194 mg/dl. Her HDL cholesterol (the "good guy") was 48 mg/dl.

Mary dived into our high-fiber prevention plan with enthusiasm. She started walking four to five miles per day and swimming a mile four times weekly. She adopted our nutrition plan for both herself and her family. By three months her blood cholesterol had dropped almost 60 points, and it has stayed under 200 for the last five years. While she has not been able to raise her HDL cholesterol (the "good guy") as high as we would like because her total cholesterol and her LDL cholesterol (the "bad guy") are so low, we are pleased with her numbers. Through

MARY'S SCORECARD				
Measurement	Initial	3 months on plan	5 years on plan	Ideal
Cholesterol, mg/dl	257	199	193	<200
LDL cholesterol, mg/dl	194	139	118	<130
HDL cholesterol, mg/dl	48	36	48	>55*
Triglycerides, mg/dl	77	118	136	<150
Exercise, miles/week	15	35	40	>20

*Goal for women ≥ 55 mg/dl, for men ≥ 45 mg/dl

our prevention diet and exercise plan she has maintained healthy values since starting the program.

Don't eat eggs. Don't eat butter. Don't eat steak. Don't eat cheese. Don't eat cake. Don't eat bacon. Most diet plans today tell us what not to eat. A continuous barrage of "don'ts" makes us feel deprived, and all too often these very foods become our next shopping list.

Do eat potatoes. Do eat pasta. Do eat squash. Do eat fresh peaches with honey. Do eat whole wheat rolls. Do eat bean burritos. We would rather tell you what to eat in this book than tell you what not to eat. So many tasty and wholesome foods are available to chose from, you shouldn't have to check your "don't" list every time you eat. If you focus on foods that are delicious and good for you most of the time, you will be able to eat anything you want.

You already know from chapter 1 that eating foods high in fiber helps prevent and treat the leading killer diseases of our time. But what you might not know is that when you eat foods high in fiber and use some common-sense principles of balance and moderation, you automatically eat a healthy diet.

A high-fiber diet is naturally low in fat, saturated fat, and cholesterol. A high-fiber diet is naturally high in complex carbohydrates, vitamins, minerals, and antioxidants. Most major health organizations today, including the American Heart Association, the American Diabetes Association, the American Dietetic Association, the American Medical Association, the American Cancer Society, and the National Academy of Sciences as well as the U.S. surgeon general, recommend this type of diet for all individuals over two years of age.

The Essence of the Prevention Plan

Our prevention plan has four components: diet, exercise, moderation, and rest and relaxation (R & R). From now on, we will call this *your* prevention plan; if you've read this far you are interested, and we'll help you get your plan rolling. Good food, regular exercise, and a healthful lifestyle including moderation and relaxation are your main defenses against chronic diseases. All of these elements improve your overall level of fitness. Better yet, they help you feel and look your best so you can enjoy life more.

Everyone should have a regular exercise program. Since walking is a great exercise that almost anyone can do, we recommend walking for most people. A *good* level, a recommended minimum, is twelve miles of walking per week. A *better* level—one we recommend for anyone with heart disease, high blood pressure, high blood cholesterol, or diabetes—is twenty miles of walking per week. The *best* level of walking, recommended for persons wanting to lose weight or maintain their weight after losing more than forty pounds, is thirty to thirty-five miles per week.

In developing your program, we recommend you count every walk of five minutes or longer. If you walk five minutes twice and ten minutes once daily, that represents about one mile. As you increase your walking your time will probably drop to fifteen minutes per mile covering four rather than three miles per hour. Walking is my main exercise, and I walk about twenty-five miles per week at thirteen to fifteen minutes per mile.

Take time to examine your lifestyle habits. If you don't smoke cigarettes, great. If you do, you'll want to stop, and we'll provide direction. If you use alcohol, do so in moderation (no more than seven drinks per week). If you are stressed out or tired, you need to get adequate rest and to start pacing your life before it outpaces you. We'll talk more in depth about exercise and lifestyle in chapter 4. This chapter will focus on your healthy eating plan.

The 1, 2, 3, 4 Food Plan

The key to good eating on your prevention plan is as easy as 1,2,3,4. Each day you should try to include in your diet *a minimum* of: *one* serving of cereal, *two* servings of fruits, *three* servings of vegetables, and *four* servings of starches. We stress that these are minimum amounts to assure that you get adequate fiber daily. Most people will need to eat more than the minimum to get enough calories. And everyone will need to round out their 1,2,3,4 plan with servings of protein foods, dairy products, fats, and other foods for a nutritionally complete and satisfying diet.

One Cereal. We recommend using cereals with at least three grams of fiber and no more than five grams of sugar per one-ounce serving (check the label). Examples of such cereals include: Fiber One, Shredded Wheat, Whole Grain Total, Whole Grain Wheaties, oat bran, and oatmeal, to name a few.

While hot and cold cereals both make a convenient and quick breakfast, they also make an excellent snack and can be combined with many foods. Many cold cereals taste good mixed with yogurt or sprinkled over fruit. Oatmeal or oat bran can be added to muffins, pancakes, casseroles, and ground-meat dishes for extra fiber.

Two Fruits. Fruits can be eaten just about anytime and require very little preparation. Try grapefruit, fresh berries, or fruit juice for breakfast; an apple, banana, or pear for lunch or snack time; and fresh pineapple, kiwi, or baked fruit for evening dessert.

Fresh fruit is the best choice, but canned, frozen, and dried fruit and fruit juices without added sugar are also good choices. Leave peelings on whenever possible to increase fiber content. One serving equals one small piece of fruit or one-half to three-quarters of a cup.

Three Vegetables. To get three servings of vegetables in daily, try eating at least one vegetable at lunch or snack time and two or more vegetables at your evening meal. Raw carrots, celery, broccoli, or cauliflower pack good in lunches and make a convenient snack. (I try to keep a container of raw cut vegetables ready in the refrigerator at all times.) One serving equals one-half cup of most vegetables and one cup of greens.

To get two servings of vegetables at your evening meal, plan both a salad and a cooked vegetable, a mixed dish containing vegetables plus a cooked vegetable or salad, or, in a pinch, eat an extra-large portion of one vegetable. As always, leave peelings on to increase fiber content.

Four Starches. Include one or more servings of bread, rolls, rice, pasta, or other starches at every meal to get in at least four servings of these foods daily. Although whole-grain starches are the best choices, refined starches such as white bread and regular pasta are also good choices.

GOOD CHOICES
white bread and rolls
soda crackers
regular pasta
wheat tortillas

BETTER CHOICES
whole-wheat bread and rolls
whole-wheat crackers
whole-wheat or spinach pasta
air-popped plain popcorn
whole-wheat tortillas
corn tortillas
white rice
wild rice

BEST CHOICES
rye or pumpernickel bread and rolls
Wasa crispbread
brown rice

You probably noticed that foods in your prevention plan include only plant foods, and that we didn't get too hung up on serving sizes. Three other types of foods—milk, meat or proteins, and fat—are also a part of a balanced and satisfying diet. But these are the foods Americans tend to overeat, adding unneeded fat and calories and contributing to chronic disease. We focus on plant foods because only plant foods contain fiber and because these are the foods Americans need to eat more of. We don't worry too much about serving sizes because when you eat enough foods with fiber, your body will tell you when to quit eating naturally.

Your prevention eating plan guarantees a minimum of 25 grams of fiber daily. We can recommend a certain number of servings from each group because foods within each group contain about the same amount of fiber.

JIM'S DIARY: For breakfast I usually eat one or two servings of oatmeal or oat bran, a banana, and skim milk. Because my father, grandfather, and several uncles died from strokes and because recent research indicates that eating one banana a day reduces risk of stroke by 50 percent, I rarely start my day without a banana.

For lunch I have a cup of raw vegetables, two oat bran muffins, twelve ounces of vegetable juice, and an orange.

Dinner begins with a very large mixed green salad with low-fat dressing. Recently I have added half an ounce of pecans (about twelve halves) to my salad since recent research indicates that four servings of nuts weekly reduce heart attack risk by 50 percent. For entrees, I eat bean burritos, pasta, broiled fish, shrimp, stir-fry chicken and vegetables over rice, pizza topped with cheese and vegetables, or vegetarian main dishes. I have two or three vegetables on the side, and my favorites are asparagus, beets, broccoli, cauliflower, and stewed tomatoes.

Dessert is usually two cups of cut-up fresh fruit. Sometimes I add sweetener, ginger, or a small amount of fat-free frozen yogurt. This pattern gives me an average of one or two cereals, four fruits, six vegetables, and four starches per weekday. I thoroughly enjoy this health-promoting eating pattern and miss it when I travel or when holidays and guests alter our habits.

Although we recommend a minimum of 25 grams of fiber daily, some people may need to eat up to the maximum of 70 grams of fiber daily to receive full benefits. Bill, my cardiology colleague, consumes over 100 grams of fiber per day, but we do not recommend this much unless you are monitored closely by your medical doctor.

High-fiber plant foods like whole grains, fruits, and vegetables taste good but are naturally low in fat and calories and are very filling. When you eat enough of these foods daily, you will find yourself eating smaller amounts of meat, dairy products, added fats, and other foods like sweets and desserts. When you focus on fiber, you won't crave too much of the high-fat foods.

Which meal would you rather eat—twelve ounces of grilled sirloin steak with black coffee and no side dishes or twelve ounces of broiled Haddock with two baked potatoes each topped with sour cream, two-thirds cup of corn, half a cup of broccoli, a lettuce salad with low-calorie dressing, one whole-grain dinner roll with butter, one scoop of ice cream, and a glass of skim milk?

The steak dinner provides no fiber while the fish dinner provides 13 grams of fiber. The steak dinner contains 1,200 calories with over 80 percent of calories from fat. The fish dinner contains 1,150 calories with less than 30 percent of the calories coming from fat.

The meal with fish contains much more food for fewer calories because it emphasizes high-fiber and low-fat foods. But if you still choose the steak, eat and enjoy it—once in a while. If you include plenty of grains, fruits, and vegetables at most meals, you can still eat your favorite high-fat foods occasionally. And if you eat a smaller portion of steak with ample high-fiber side dishes, so much the better.

Unless you are trying to lose weight in a hurry (see chapter 3 if you are), you won't need to worry about how much food you eat. When you follow the prevention plan, your body will automatically tell you when to quit eating.

Unique Bean-ifits

Dried beans, lentils, and peas are nutritionally unique and deserve special mention. Beans are an excellent source of protein, vitamins, and minerals. They can substitute for meat in many dishes. Beans are also a great source of fiber and are particularly rich in soluble fiber—the kind of fiber that helps control blood fat levels.

Commonly used dried beans include pinto, navy, lima, garbanzo, black beans, black-eyed peas, and lentils. Adding one-half cup serving of cooked dried beans to your 1,2,3,4 plan will add 8 grams of fiber to your daily diet.

JIM'S DIARY: Bean burritos are one of my favorite entrees and I usually eat them about twice a week. Try my bean burrito recipe (see the recipe section). In addition, I usually have canned beans once or twice a week. I often open a can of pork and beans, dip out the chunk of pork fat and add barbecue sauce or salsa for a quick and tasty lunch. Usually I have pinto or navy beans or black-eyed peas for lunch at the cafeteria on Sunday. At a salad bar, I always take at least one-half cup of garbanzo or kidney beans. One of my favorite canned beans is Trappey's jalapeño black-eyed peas, which I have for lunch with stewed tomatoes. While I don't eat beans every single day of the week, I average more than seven servings per week.

We recommend that you follow my pattern and eat a serving of cooked or canned dried beans as often as possible, preferably up to seven one-half cup servings weekly. Try them—you'll like them.

An Overall Balance

Of course, the fiber-containing plant foods are not the only foods you'll eat each day. But if you eat the right amount of these foods, you'll find it much easier to keep an overall balance in your diet.

The 1,2,3,4 plan is not intended to be your entire diet but to assure that you get adequate fiber daily. Your total diet should also include two servings of low-fat dairy products (three to four for teenagers and for women who are pregnant or breastfeeding), four to six ounces of lean meat or other protein food (beans!) daily, and a modest amount of fat from salad dressings and oils. You don't need to search out fat to include in your daily diet because the fat will find you. My patients tell me that ice cream and cookies call their name. Certainly the cookie shop at the exit of the cafeteria and the vending machines at the hospital know my name.

The U.S. Department of Agriculture recently introduced its new "Food Guide Pyramid." The food pyramid pictures bread, cereal, rice, and pasta as the foundation of an upright pyramid, followed by fruits and vegetables in the middle and dairy products, proteins foods, and added fats at the top.

The aim of our prevention plan is consistent with that of the food pyramid: we want you to build your diet on high-fiber plant foods and top it with smaller amounts of dairy products, meats, and added fats. These "topping" foods are important sources of protein and many vitamins and minerals in our American diet. But they also contain greater amounts of fat, saturated fat, cholesterol, and calories than plant foods and can contribute to killer diseases if eaten in excess.

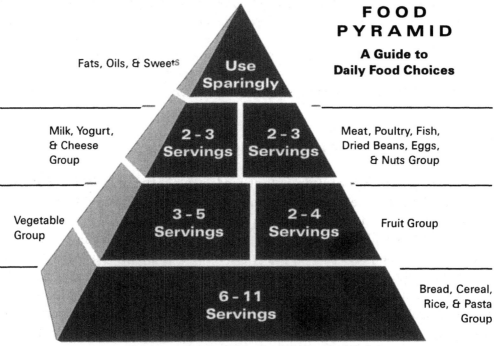

FOOD PYRAMID

A Guide to Daily Food Choices

Fats, Oils, & Sweets

Use Sparingly

Milk, Yogurt, & Cheese Group

2 - 3 Servings

2 - 3 Servings

Meat, Poultry, Fish, Dried Beans, Eggs, & Nuts Group

Vegetable Group

3 - 5 Servings

2 - 4 Servings

Fruit Group

6 - 11 Servings

Bread, Cereal, Rice, & Pasta Group

Source: U.S. Department of Agriculture, U.S. Department of Health and Human Services

Don't Chew the Fat

Fats in the diet fall into three main categories. Saturated fats are saturated with hydrogen and contain no double bonds between the carbon atom components. Saturated fats are animal fats like butter, lard, and the marbling around meat, which are solid at room temperature. Saturated fats raise blood cholesterol, promote hardening of the arteries, and contribute to blood clots that clog blood vessels to the heart and brain resulting in heart attacks and strokes.

Monounsaturated fats have a single double bond between two carbon atoms. Olive oil and canola oil are rich in monounsaturates and are liquid at room temperature. These may be the healthiest oils to add to your diet in salad dressing and when stir-frying.

Polyunsaturated fats have two or more double bonds between carbon atoms. Most vegetable oils and fish oils are polyunsaturates, which are also liquid at room temperature. To make stick margarines and shortening, food manufacturers expose vegetable oils to hydrogen to hydrogenate them and eliminate double bonds. These hydrogenated oils resemble saturated fats from animal products and have the same adverse health effects on blood cholesterol and blood vessels.

Cholesterol is only found in animal products. Some vegetable oils and shortenings used to advertise that they were cholesterol free. While this claim was true, it was misleading because some consumers concluded that these 100 percent fat products were healthful. In fact, the less fat of any type we eat the healthier we tend to be. Japanese and Chinese people who lived on only 10 percent of calories from fat had extremely low rates of heart disease. So even if you are using olive oil or vegetable oil, use it sparingly.

Animal foods also contain more fats than plant foods. Fats provide twice the calories per equal weight unit that carbohydrates or proteins do (9 calories per gram for fat compared to 4 calories per gram for carbohydrate or protein), so high-fat foods contain much more calories than high-carbohydrate or high-protein foods.

Americans get 42 percent of their daily fat intake from meat, poultry, and fish, 17 percent from dairy products, and 10 percent from added fats and sweets. In contrast, Americans get 15 percent of their daily fat intake from grain products (and this figure includes cakes, pies, cookies, and pastries!) and 9 percent from fruits and vegetables.

All major health organizations today recommend that Americans over two years of age get no more than 30 percent of their calories as fat. Because our prevention plan is rich in carbohydrate-containing plant foods, you should find it easy to control your fat intake. When you use the recipes in this book, you won't need to worry about fat content, because all our recipes contain less than 30 percent of calories as fat.

Although many animal foods are higher in fat, saturated fat, and cholesterol than plant foods, animal foods are especially rich in certain vitamins and minerals and play an important role in good nutrition. Dairy products are a great source of calcium and protein. Meats are rich in protein, niacin, iron, and thiamin. You don't need to eliminate meat and dairy products from your diet—just choose the kind, quantity, and preparation techniques carefully.

Choose nonfat dairy products like skim milk, nonfat yogurt, and nonfat frozen yogurt for your prevention plan. You won't miss the extra fat and cholesterol, and you'll still get all the calcium and vitamins and minerals of whole dairy products.

Choose leaner cuts of red meat such as round, sirloin, loin, flank, or extra-lean ground beef, and pork loin, tenderloin, fresh ham, or Canadian bacon. Trim all visible fat before cooking and bake, broil, boil, or grill rather than fry when possible. If you do fry, fry in nonstick cookware or use vegetable oil spray.

Use fish and seafood often since they have unique nutritional benefits. Use poultry moderately since it has less fat than red meat. Be sure to remove the skin before cooking. You will find that your fish, seafood, and poultry are tastiest if broiled to the juicy just-done stage rather than fried or cooked to death.

A COMPARISON OF DIETARY FATS

Type of Oil	Cholesterol mg/tbls	Saturated Fat	Polyunsaturated Fat	Other Fats	Monounsaturated Fat
Crisco Puritan Oil (canola)	0	6	31	1	62
Crisco Vegetable Oil	0	10	51	0	39
Crisco Corn Canola Oil	0	10	47	0	43
Safflower Oil	0	9	78	1	12
Sunflower Oil	0	11	69	0	20
Corn Oil	0	13	62	0	25
Peanut Oil	0	13	33	5	49
Olive Oil	0	14	9	0	77
Soybean Oil (vegetable)	0	15	61	0	24
Margarine (fat)	0	18	29	5	48
Vegetable Shortening	0	25	25	7	43
Cottonseed Oil	0	27	54	0	19
Chicken Fat	11	30	22	1	47
Lard	12	41	12	0	47
Animal Fat Shortening	9	43	6	3	48
Beef Fat	14	52	3	1	44
Palm Oil	0	51	10	0	39
Butter (fat)	33	55	3	12	30
Coconut Oil	0	77	2	15	6

JIM'S DIARY: At breakfast and lunch I usually stick to grains, vegetables, beans, and fruits. For the evening meal, I like to eat fish or seafood twice weekly, chicken or turkey once or twice weekly, lean red meat two or three times monthly, pasta with cheese weekly and a vegetarian meal once or twice weekly. At the cafeteria on Sunday I eat vegetarian and on our Friday night out I usually order fish, pasta, a bean burrito, or an Oriental seafood dish.

If you prefer to eat vegetarian-style all the time, fine. Combining any two of three plant groups—beans, nuts and seeds, and grains—yields complete, high-quality protein. Vegetarians have lower fat and calories intakes and lower rates of almost all major chronic diseases than nonvegetarians. But it's not necessary to eat vegetarian to achieve the benefits of our prevention plan if you still emphasize plant foods in your diet.

Sweets, desserts, and added fats such as butter, margarine, and salad dressings contribute little nutritionally to our diet but enhance eating pleasure and satisfaction. No one should have to give these foods up. Again, it's a matter of choices, quantities, and frequency.

Choose soft margarine over butter (better yet, jam, jelly, or other seasonings), vegetable oils (especially olive or canola oil, which are rich in monounsaturated fat) over solid shortening or meat drippings, and low-fat or reduced-calorie salad dressings over mayonnaise or regular salad dressings. Look for the term "hydrogenated" or "partially hydrogenated" on the labels of products since the health benefits of these vegetable oils are lost when they are hydrogenated.

Choose fruit-based or high-sugar desserts over high-fat ones. Believe it or not, sugar is the lesser of the two evils, because sugar is a carbohydrate (and, remember, carbohydrates contain 4 calories per gram whereas fats contain 9 calories per gram).

One-half cup of sliced sugared strawberries over a slice of angel food cake topped with two tablespoons of whipped topping contains only 158 calories and 2 grams of fat, compared to the 238 calories and 13 grams of fat in a two-by-two inch slice of strawberry cheesecake.

Use salt sparingly, and experiment with seasonings and spices to enhance the natural flavor of foods. Bay leaves, dry mustard, marjoram, nutmeg, pepper, and vegetables such as onions, green peppers, and mushrooms
go well with beef; lemon, marjoram, paprika, parsley, sage, and thyme go
well with poultry; and apples, garlic, onion, and sage go good with pork.
Lemon, onion, and vinegar can enhance the natural flavor of vegetables.

Gift from the Sea

Scientists have known for years that heart disease is almost nonexistent
in Eskimos and other populations who eat large quantities of oily fish.
Only recently, however, have researchers discovered a possible reason for
this finding.

Fish are in a special class as far as protein foods go. Not only do fish
contain less fat and calories than most red meats, but the small amount
of fat in fish is made up of a unique class of fatty acids called the omega-3
fatty acids.

The omega-3 fats are one of the few unsaturated fats found in foods
of animal origin. Many studies show that omega-3 fats lower blood triglyceride (a kind of fat) levels dramatically and blood cholesterol levels
modestly in individuals with high initial levels. Omega-3 fats also pro-
long blood clotting time, thus preventing blood clots in blood vessels and
reducing risk for heart attacks and strokes.

We recommend that you try to eat fish twice weekly for their omega-
3 fat content. More oily fishes like salmon, mackerel, haddock, trout, and
herring contain more of these omega-3 fats. Sardines are an especially
rich source of omega-3 fats.

Besides getting the benefits of this special class of fats, you will also
benefit from the fewer calories in fish. Six ounces of broiled cod contains
only 178 calories and about 1 gram of fat, compared to the 377 calories
and 26 grams of fat in a six-ounce T-bone steak.

Be careful, though, not to sabotage your healthy fish choice by adding a lot of fat in cooking. Poached, steamed, broiled, or grilled fish with lemon is both delicious and healthy.

JIM'S DIARY: As I said earlier, I eat fish or seafood about twice weekly because this has the potential to reduce heart attack risk by 50 percent. I used to eat sardines daily, but this was expensive and gave me extra calories. Now, because my blood triglycerides tend to be a little high, I take two fish oil capsules daily. Since I started doing this my triglycerides have decreased from about 330 mg/dl to about 80 mg/dl. If your triglyceride level is above 250 mg/dl you may want to ask your doctor about the use of fish oil capsules.

Emphasizing Soluble Fiber

Fiber is grouped into two broad categories—soluble and insoluble. Soluble fiber has the greater cholesterol-lowering effect, while insoluble fiber is more effective for improving bowel function. Both types of fiber help regulate blood sugar.

Most foods contain a mix of both soluble and insoluble fiber, but some foods contain more of one type than the other. Dried beans, oatmeal and oat bran, psyllium, and some fruits and vegetables are especially rich sources of soluble fiber. Wheat bran and most other grains are good sources of insoluble fiber.

Both types of fiber are important for overall health, and you should try to eat a variety of fruits, vegetables, and grains daily for a good fiber balance. If you have a problem with high blood fat levels, however, we recommend that you try to emphasize foods high in soluble fiber.

Oats and dried beans and peas are two of the best food sources of soluble fiber. Other foods rich in soluble fiber include barley and several fruits and vegetables.

JIM'S DIARY: For my own high blood cholesterol problem, I try to eat one bowl of oat cereal and two oat bran muffins, one-half to one cup of cooked dried beans, or a combination of these foods daily. This gives me about 7 or 8 grams of soluble fiber from these sources alone.

What about Supplements?

To achieve the benefits of our prevention plan, you need to eat at least 25 grams of fiber from food daily. That's because other things in your diet—fat, saturated fat, cholesterol, and calories—count, and high-fiber intake helps control these.

But for persons who have high blood cholesterol levels that do not respond adequately to diet, we often recommend a fiber supplement such as psyllium (in sugar-free Metamucil) in addition to a high-fiber diet. However, such steps should be taken only under the advice of your doctor. For most of us, a high-fiber diet will bring down cholesterol levels nicely and will provide other health benefits as well.

Our prevention plan is rich in nutrient-dense foods—foods that provide a lot of vitamins and minerals for few calories. If you follow the 1,2,3,4 plan, round it out with servings from the milk and meat or protein group and eat a variety of foods in each group, you probably will not need to take vitamin and mineral supplements. However, the only disadvantage of taking a multiple vitamin and mineral supplement, such as Thera M, is the expense. Many people are beginning to take supplemental antioxidants—beta carotene, vitamin C, and vitamin E. While a certain level of vitamins and minerals is good for your body, too much is not and is also a waste of money.

Timing

Our research shows that spreading your fiber intake throughout the day has a greater effect on health than taking it mostly in one meal. Spreading your fiber throughout the day will also help to raise your satiety level and tell your body how much other food you need.

When we first started recommending our diet back in the 1970s, people were amazed at the quantity and variety of foods they could eat. Many of them could not eat everything because they were too full. If you are not used to eating many fiber-containing foods such as fruits, vegetables, or grains, build up to your 25 grams or more of fiber gradually—perhaps over a few weeks. This will give your system time to adjust to the larger fiber intake gradually and will prevent the bloating or gas that can occasionally come with drastic changes in fiber intake. Be sure to drink plenty of fluids also.

When should you start on your high-fiber prevention plan? Why delay the pleasures and benefits of good eating? Begin today!

Chapter Action Plan

Goal
- Start with *one* cereal
- Enjoy *two* fruits
- Include *three* vegetables
- Add *four* starches
- Eat dried beans *several* times weekly
- Have fish *twice* weekly

I Can Do That!
- Figure out about how many servings of cereals, fruits, vegetables, starches, beans, and fish you eat now.
- For those foods not yet at goal level, increase the number of servings by one. For example, if you only eat one serving of vegetables daily now, push for two.
- If you never eat dried beans now, start by trying them once weekly.
- Gradually build up your number of servings until you reach your prevention plan goal.

Prevention Notes

• A banana a day can cut risk for stroke by 50 percent.

• Four servings of nuts per week can reduce risk for heart attack by 50 percent.
   Tree nuts, such as pecans, are better than ground nuts, such as peanuts.

• Two servings of fish per week can reduce risk for heart attack by 50 percent.

MY PREVENTION FOOD PLAN			
Food	**Ideal**	**Now I eat:**	**Goal for next week:**
Cereal	1 / day	___ / day	___ / day
Fruit	2 / day	___ / day	___ / day
Vegetables	3 / day	___ / day	___ / day
Starches	4 / day	___ / day	___ / day
Beans	3 / week	___ / week	___ / week
Fish	2 / week	___ / week	___ / week

3
YOUR QUICK LOSS PLAN

SUCCESS STORY:
Ann drops her weight and blood cholesterol.

Ann, a fifty-three-year-old housewife, came to see me because she had high blood cholesterol, high blood pressure, and she was overweight. She walked about five miles per week. She was 5 feet, 4 inches tall, weighed 210 pounds, and had a blood pressure of 160/100 and a blood cholesterol of 338 mg/dl. We counseled her to increase her walking and begin our quick loss plan with a goal of losing about one to two pounds per week.

Ann eagerly adopted our recommendations and surprised us with a weight loss of nineteen pounds in the first month. Her blood pressure and cholesterol level also plummeted. Over the next nine months we saw her every four to six weeks and she continued to exercise, follow the diet, and lose weight. At ten months she was walking forty minutes on the treadmill six times weekly. Her weight was 160 pounds, her blood pressure was 130/70, and her cholesterol was 263 mg/dl. We had to add some medicine to lower cholesterol into an acceptable range. She continues to follow our diet and exercise program.

ANN'S SCORECARD				
Measurement	Initial	1 month on plan	3 months on plan	10 months on plan
Weight, lbs.	212	193	181	160
Blood Pressure	160/100	136/106	130/82	130/70
Cholesterol, mg/dl	338	263	233	263
Triglycerides, mg/dl	234	166	173	224
Exercise, miles/week	4	6	10	16

When we first started using high-fiber diets for our patients with diabetes, not only did the condition of our patients improve dramatically, but our patients' spouses lost weight unintentionally. Maria lost more than ten pounds when her dentist husband started our prevention diet to manage his diabetes. When I first started experimenting with oat bran to lower my own cholesterol level, I lost eight pounds in five weeks without trying. In many of our research studies with high-fiber diets, our participants lose weight on diets providing the amount of calories calculated to maintain their weight. Fiber clearly promotes weight loss.

Our quick weight loss plan is as easy as 1, 2, 3: eat a low-calorie diet that is high in fiber and low in fat, walk at least twelve miles per week with a goal of twenty to thirty-five miles, and keep a diary of all the food you eat and the calories you burn with exercise.

A high-fiber diet combined with regular exercise and a healthful lifestyle is the ideal weight loss route for most people. High-fiber diets are low in calories, low in fat, yet high in volume. You'd be surprised how much good food you can eat on a 1,200-calorie high-fiber diet.

Consider the following 1,200-calorie daily menu: 1 cup Cheerios, ¾ cup blueberries, 1 cup skim milk, ½ whole-grain English muffin, and 1 tablespoon light margarine for breakfast; 2½ cups salad with lettuce, carrots, zucchini, tomato, and 2 tablespoons dressing, 4 slices melba toast, and 1 cup skim milk for lunch; 6 ounces baked fish, ½ cup lima beans, ½ cup broccoli, 1 small roll and 1 tablespoon light margarine for dinner; and 3 cups air-popped popcorn for a snack.

Now compare this to a traditional 1,200-calorie diet menu, which might look like this: 2 slices toast with 2 teaspoons jam for breakfast; 1 slice bread with 1 ounce of meat, 1 ounce of cheese, and 1 teaspoon mayonnaise, and 1 cup 2 percent milk for lunch; a 4-ounce hamburger patty, ¼ cup cottage cheese, 1 peach half, a lettuce leaf, and 1 cup 2 percent milk for dinner; and no snacks. Which menu do you think you think would be more satisfying?

If you don't have that much weight to lose or aren't in a hurry to lose it, following our regular prevention plan will help you lose weight the best way—slowly and easily. But if you want to lose weight fast or have weight-related health problems that require quicker weight loss, we recommend our quick loss plan.

We have used our quick loss plan with hundreds of patients since 1974. Here are two more examples:

SUCCESS STORY:
Susan decreases weight and blood cholesterol.

Susan was a twenty-seven-year-old sales associate who came to see me because of high blood cholesterol and a strong family history of heart disease. Her father died at age thirty of his third heart attack. Her father's uncle awaited a heart transplant at age forty-nine after his first heart attack at age thirty-nine and bypass surgery at age forty. Susan previously tried a conventional low-fat diet with little success.

Susan measured 5 feet, 1 inch tall and weighed 130 pounds—about twenty pounds more than her ideal weight. Her blood cholesterol was 257 mg/dl and her blood triglycerides were 156 mg/dl. Susan regularly walked four to five miles weekly.

Because of her threatening family history, we started Susan on our 1,200-calorie quick loss plan. Over the next few weeks Susan followed the plan faithfully and increased her walking to ten miles weekly. In the next two weeks Susan lost four pounds and dropped her cholesterol to 208 mg/dl and her triglycerides to 131 mg/dl—down 19 percent for cholesterol and 16 percent for triglycerides.

Two months later we saw Susan again. By now she had built up to nearly eighteen miles of walking weekly and lost sixteen pounds—down to 114 pounds. Her blood cholesterol was 199 mg/dl and her blood triglycerides were 151 mg/dl. Her level of artery-clogging low-density lipoprotein cholesterol continues to drop from initial levels, while her level of protective high-density lipoprotein cholesterol are shooting up.

SUCCESS STORY:
Rick lowers weight and insulin needs.

Rick was forty-four years old when he first came to see me. He had developed diabetes six years before and was now taking 55 units of insulin daily, with persistent poor blood sugar control. His blood pressure was high at 160/90 mm Hg (millimeters of mercury), though he was not taking medication for this. He weighed 238 pounds—over sixty pounds above what he should weight at 5 feet, 11 inches. His blood fat levels had crept dangerously high—296 mg/dl for cholesterol and 936 mg/dl for triglycerides.

We started Rick on our 1,600-calorie quick loss plan and a walking program that included two miles of walking daily. We also advised Rick to cut his insulin dose to 40 units daily, since insulin requirements usually fall with both exercise and a diet.

Two weeks later Rick returned to our office and reported following the plan effortlessly. His weight had dropped seven pounds and his blood pressure had fallen to 132/74 mm Hg. His blood sugar control had improved, and we were able to lower his daily insulin dose to 25 units.

We talked to Rick on the telephone at frequent intervals and saw him again seven weeks later. He had lost another fourteen pounds and maintained a normal blood pressure. At this time we re-measured his blood fat levels. His blood cholesterol had fallen 124 points to 172 mg/dl, and his triglycerides had plummeted 773 points. His blood sugar remained in good control on the lower insulin dose.

Rick's weight, blood pressure, blood sugar control, and blood fat levels continued to improve over the next ten weeks as we gradually weaned Rick off insulin.

Six months after starting the prevention plan, Rick continued to walk eighteen to twenty miles weekly and had lost a total of thirty pounds. He no longer had high blood pressure and no longer needed insulin to maintain his blood sugar in the safe range of under 150 mg/dl. His blood cholesterol was 188 mg/dl, and his triglycerides were 167 mg/dl—both perfectly healthy.

The quick loss plan helps people lose weight easily and keep it off, since it teaches the foundation for healthful, high-fiber eating for the future.

What Is the Quick Loss Plan?

The quick loss plan is a low-calorie, low-fat, but high-fiber eating plan designed to get the pounds off quickly. It is really just a more structured form of our regular prevention plan—the bare bones prevention plan with specific advice on food servings for those who want detailed guidance on what to eat.

Once you have lost weight, you will want to continue to eat in the 1,2,3,4 pattern (one cereal, two fruits, three vegetables, and four starches daily) without worrying about exact amounts or extras. Of course, you'll also want to maintain your regular exercise routine and maintain a low fat intake.

We present your quick loss plan at two different calorie levels—one geared more for women and one geared more for men. Many women are eating between 1,800 and 2,200 calories daily to maintain their current body weight. Cutting the calories to about 1,200 daily will help most women lose one to two pounds weekly.

Unfair as it may seem, men have more bone and muscle and therefore require more calories than most women. Many men are maintaining their current body weight by consuming 2,200 to 2,600 calories daily and will lose one to two pounds weekly on about 1,600 calories.

The quick loss plan provides about 25 to 30 percent of calories as fat, 50 to 55 percent as carbohydrate, and 15 to 20 percent of calories as protein. The 1,200-calorie plan provides about 30 grams of fiber, whereas the 1600-calorie plan provides about 40 to 45 grams.

Who Is the Quick Loss Plan For?

The quick loss plan is for anyone who has thirty or more pounds to lose or who needs to lose weight quickly. Generally we recommend the quick loss plan for individuals who have significant weight-related health problems or for individuals who weigh at least 20 percent more than they should. We do not recommend the quick loss plan for individuals over seventy years of age unless they have significant medical reasons for quick weight loss.

You can get an idea of the body weight right for you by using the following quick formula. MALES: Allow 106 pounds for the first five feet of your height plus six pounds for each extra inch. FEMALES: Allow 100

DESIRABLE BODY WEIGHTS*				
Height	Men		Women	
	Ideal	Obese	Ideal	Obese
4' 10"			115	138
4' 11"			117	140
5'			120	144
5' 1"			122	146
5' 2"	136	163	125	150
5' 3"	138	166	128	154
5' 4"	140	168	131	157
5' 5"	143	172	134	161
5' 6"	145	174	137	164
5' 7"	148	178	140	168
5' 8"	151	181	143	172
5' 9"	154	185	146	175
5' 10"	157	188	149	179
5' 11"	160	192	152	182
6'	164	197	155	186
6' 1"	167	201		
6' 2"	171	205		
6' 3"	175	210		
6' 4"	179	215		

*Ideal weights are the mid-points for weight for medium frame from the 1983 Metropolitan Height and Weight Tables (JAMA 260:2548, 1988). Obese weights are calculated at more than 20 percent above the ideal weight.

pounds for the first five feet of your height plus five pounds for each extra inch.

Height and weight tables can also serve as a body-weight guide. Depending on your frame size, build, and amount of muscle, a good weight for you might be more or less than weights listed in these tables.

Assess your need to lose weight realistically. Goal weights should be more generous for older persons. Newspapers, magazines, and television shows today often set unrealistic weight ideals for society. Over one-half of the adult population in this country went on diets last year, and nearly 90 percent of Americans think they weigh too much. Most of us can't and shouldn't try to look like the models we see in magazines. A large percentage of women feel they are too heavy although they are at a healthy weight. Instead of worrying about your appearance, we'd like for you to think of your body weight in terms of health consequences.

Excess body fat aggravates heart disease, diabetes, stroke, cancer, and high blood pressure. If you have a problem with any of these diseases and are overweight, losing weight will probably greatly improve your symptoms and may even eliminate your disease. For some people, losing weight is the single most important therapy.

For some people, a desirable body weight seems hopelessly far away. Don't despair! You don't have to get to an ideal weight to benefit from weight loss. Losing even fifteen to twenty pounds can improve blood pressure, diabetes, arthritis, and can lessen problems from heart disease. And if your ultimate goal is larger, set small, realistic weight loss goals to move you toward your eventual goal. You'll find that if you adopt a high-fiber eating style, weight loss will come naturally and easily.

Why Does the Quick Loss Plan Work?

The quick loss plan works effortlessly because high-fiber foods take longer to eat, fill you up, and contain fewer calories than low-fiber foods. Three slices of whole-wheat toast with one teaspoon of raspberry jam on each provides fewer calories than one chocolate eclair. One ten-ounce bag of plain frozen broccoli provides fewer calories than two homemade sugar cookies.

Which snack would you feel more satisfied after, a large apple or one-third of a glass of apple juice? The large apple contains almost 4 grams of fiber and would take the average person about ten to fifteen minutes to munch. The apple juice contains no fiber and would take the average person ten to fifteen seconds to guzzle down.

We tested hunger and satiety levels in men on two different 800-calorie diets—one high in fiber and one low in fiber. When the men ate the high-fiber diet, they consistently reported greater satiety and less hunger after all meals and before the noon and evening meals. Another study showed that people felt more satisfied on a high-fiber diet containing half as many calories as a lower fiber diet.

Studies consistently show that high-fiber foods and diets curb appetite and boost satiety. Foods high in fiber take longer to leave the stomach, leaving us feeling fuller longer. They also lower blood levels of insulin, an appetite-stimulating hormone. Finally, by-products of fiber breakdown in the gut may also suppress appetite.

Calories In, Calories Out

As difficult as it is for most people, weight loss boils down to a simple equation between calories in and calories out. If you eat more calories than you burn, you gain weight. If you burn more calories than you eat, you lose weight.

New research indicates that the fat you eat promotes fat accumulation much more than does sugar, starch, and protein. Remember that carbohydrates and protein contain only 4 calories per gram, while fat contains 9 calories per gram. High-fiber foods are usually high in carbohydrate, low in fat, and therefore low in calories. Nutrients such as starch may also be less available to the body in high-fiber foods, lowering the effective calorie content of these foods even further.

When we emphasize fiber in our diet, we work on the *calories in* side of the equation—lowering the amount of calories we eat each day. The flip side of the equation, *calories out*, is equally important. People in the United States today burn 75 percent fewer calories in physical activity than they did a century ago. A farmer in the 1900s walked the equivalent of 120 miles weekly doing farm chores. It took his 125-pound wife more than two hours and 200 calories just to prepare daily dinner for the family.

Try to boost the calories you burn each day any way you can. Regular exercise such as a half hour of walking daily not only burns calories but improves heart health, muscle tone, energy level, and mental outlook. I find that when I exercise regularly, I don't feel like overeating.

Be more active throughout your day as well. Park your car farther away from work and walk a few extra blocks. Take the stairs instead of the elevator. (Ten minutes of stair climbing burns two to three times as many calories as ten minutes of walking.) Try to develop active hobbies such as gardening, woodworking, bowling, or tennis. These activities get us up and moving, away from the television and away from the refrigerator.

Why Are Records Important?

Keeping records of all your food intake and all your exercise calories is essential for sustained weight loss and long-term management. Yes, I said *essential*. We have treated over one thousand obese individuals in the University of Kentucky Weight Management Program and found three fundamental practices for successful weight loss and weight management: keeping accurate food and exercise records, walking at least twenty miles per week, and eating a high-fiber, low-fat diet.

JIM'S DIARY: My father was 5 feet, 2 inches tall and weighed 230 pounds before he had a stroke at age forty-one. He used to cut the fat from a piece of ham or steak and relish eating it at the end of the main course, before dessert. I grew up on good southern cooking with bacon or sausage, biscuits, and brown gravy for breakfast; bologna and cheese sandwiches with cookies for lunch; and a full course dinner of pork chops or chicken-fried steak, potatoes, gravy, and, always, dessert.

I inherited a love of food, sweets, and fat from my dad. My mother taught me to enjoy and cook these tasty high-fat foods. These habits led to my tendency to be overweight and have high blood cholesterol.

At 5 feet, 8 inches tall, I have weighed as much as 189 pounds—at least twenty-five pounds more than my doctor advises me to weigh. In 1986 I did lose down to 155 pounds and now am working to keep my weight in a reasonable zone. To do this I have kept records of my food intake, exercise, and fruit and vegetable intake for the last two years. You're right—that's a lot of effort. But I have learned after twenty-five years of struggling with extra weight that I need this discipline to keep my eating in check and to promote the healthful practices of exercise and fruit and vegetable use.

To keep track of your food intake and exercise output, buy a three-by-five inch spiral notebook and carry it with you at all times. Write down everything that goes in your mouth and record all your exercise. To estimate your exercise calories, use the following formula. Walking one mile burns 100 calories if you weigh 150 pounds. If you weigh 120 pounds, you burn 120/150 or 0.8 x 100 = 80 calories per mile. If you weigh 210 pounds, you burn 210/150 or 1.4 x 100 = 140 calories per mile.

Avoiding the Yo-Yo Syndrome

The goal of weight loss for all of us is to keep it off permanently. People who lose and then regain large amounts of weight may actually be worse off healthwise than if they had never lost weight to begin with. And once you have regained lost weight, you may find it harder to lose weight the next time.

To keep weight off permanently, you must permanently change whatever it was that made you gain weight. For most people, diet, activity, and behavior patterns all contribute to weight gain.

After you have slimmed down on our quick loss plan, adopt our 1,2,3,4 prevention plan for life. When you eat enough grains, fruits, vegetables, and legumes, no foods are off-limits, and your body will be able to tell you when to stop eating. You won't feel restricted, and you won't have to continually keep track of every little bite you eat.

Of all lifestyle and eating behaviors studied, the one that best predicts whether you will keep your weight off is whether you exercise regularly. If you keep up regular walking, jogging, aerobics, or some other vigorous exercise for a lifetime, your chances of keeping your weight off improve dramatically. If your schedule is hectic, choose a form of exercise that slips comfortably into your daily routine.

JIM'S DIARY: In attempting to keep my boyish figure I need to walk at least twenty miles per week. Over the last two years I have kept a log of my daily exercise and have averaged twenty-five miles of walking per week. I walk a fifteen-minute mile comfortably and under race conditions can cover 6.2 miles with a walk-jog routine in less than seventy-four minutes, or under twelve minutes per mile. Each day I park a mile away from the hospital and thus force myself to walk at least two miles per day. I make rounds and see patients in two hospitals and two different clinic buildings and sometimes log more than ten miles daily by walking everywhere and taking the stairs. I walk about a mile to the faculty club once weekly for lunch while some of my colleagues drive. If I have had a slow week I often walk four to six miles on weekends. In nice weather I occasionally walk four miles to work. When I travel I always have comfortable walking shoes and frequently am able to walk two miles between connections while waiting in the airport. In most cities I walk to restaurants and frequently will walk six to eight miles while sightseeing. I enjoy walking but must keep a careful log to ensure that I get in at least twenty-five miles per week.

A Daily Plan

The quick loss plan is a balanced and safe weight loss diet for adults. Children and women who are pregnant or breastfeeding have special nutritional needs and should not follow this plan.

If you are a woman, we recommend that you follow the 1,200-calorie plan. If you are a man, we recommend that you follow the 1,600-calorie plan. Of course, men can follow the 1,200-calorie plan if they want to lose weight faster, but remember that the more restricted your diet is, the less likely you are to follow it. You can follow the quick loss plan as long as you need to lose your unwanted pounds. If you follow the 1,200-calorie plan, we recommend that you take a low-dose multivitamin and mineral tablet daily such as a Thera M preparation. No matter how nutritious your food choices are, it's hard to get in all the vitamins and minerals you need on 1,200 calories.

Chapter Action Plan

Goal

- Follow a high-fiber, nutritious diet (1,200 or 1,600 calories).
- Exercise regularly (walk twelve, twenty, or thirty to thirty-five miles per week).
- Keep records of all food and exercise.

I Can Do That!

- Purchase a three-by-five inch spiral notebook.
- Record your exercise and *all* the food you eat.
- To start with, increase your walking by 50 percent or six miles (whichever is the least).
- Start on the 1,200- or 1,600-calorie diet plan. (See the sample menus on the next two pages.)

SAMPLE 1,200-CALORIE MENU	
Food Examples	**Food Category**
BREAKFAST	
¾ cup oat bran cold cereal	1 serving cereal
½ banana, sliced	1 serving fruit
1 cup skim milk	1 serving milk
coffee or tea	free
NOON MEAL	
½ cup vegetable sticks	1 serving vegetables
½ cup baked beans	1 serving beans
6 small rye crackers	1 serving starch
1 small apple	1 serving fruit
iced tea, diet cola, or mineral water	free
EVENING MEAL	
2 cups mixed greens	1 serving vegetables
1 tablespoon low-fat dressing	1 serving fat
8 ounces broiled fish	4 servings protein
½ cup beets	1 serving vegetables
1 small boiled potato	1 serving starch
1 small whole-wheat roll	1 serving starch
1 tablespoon light margarine	1 serving fat
5 ounces low-fat yogurt with	
1 packet sweetener	1 serving milk
decaffeinated coffee or tea	free
SNACK	
3 cups air-popped popcorn	1 serving starch
MISCELLANEOUS	
2 teaspoons canola oil (for use anytime during day in cooking or on salads)	2 servings fat

SAMPLE 1,600-CALORIE MENU	
Food Examples	**Food Category**
BREAKFAST	
1 cup strawberries	1 serving fruit
3 ounces low-fat yogurt with	½ serving milk
1 packet sweetener	
2 oat muffins	3 servings starch
1 tablespoon light margarine	1 serving fat
coffee or tea	free
NOON MEAL	
4 ounces vegetable juice	1 serving vegetables
2 slices whole-wheat bread	2 servings starch
2 ounces sliced turkey breast	2 servings protein
1 medium pear	2 servings fruit
iced tea, diet cola, or mineral water	free
EVENING MEAL	
2 cups garden salad with	1 serving vegetables
½ cup garbanzo beans	1 serving beans
2 tablespoons low-fat dressing	2 servings fat
4 ounces baked chicken	4 servings protein
½ cup green beans	1 serving vegetables
1 serving oven "fried potatoes"	1 serving starch
½ cup stewed tomatoes	1 serving vegetables
½ cup blueberries	1 serving fruit
3 ounces frozen nonfat yogurt	1 serving milk
decaffeinated coffee or tea	free
SNACK	
¾ cup Nutrigrain cereal	1 serving cereal
½ cup skim milk	½ serving milk
MISCELLANEOUS	
2 teaspoons canola oil (for use anytime during the day in cooking or on salads)	2 servings fat

4
HEALTHFUL LIVING

SUCCESS STORY:
Barry is energized by jogging.

Barry was a sixty-three-year-old college professor. He felt tired and worn out much of the time and attributed these feelings to his advancing age. He sometimes had difficulty concentrating and next found himself taking occasional catnaps at work.

Barry thought it was time to retire. Then on an impulse Barry decided to try something new to him. Barry had never been a regular exerciser before, but he talked to his doctor and decided to start a walking program. Barry began slowly, since he hadn't done much more than routine yard work for several years. After a month or so of walking, Barry began to notice he had more energy and was not so continually sleepy. Barry became enthused about how the walking was helping him and decided to step up his exercise program to slow jogging.

Four years later Barry is still hooked on exercise. At age sixty-seven, Barry now jogs about five miles at least five times weekly. He no longer falls asleep on the job and says he has more energy now than he did ten or even twenty years ago. Barry even ran in a marathon.

You and I don't have to run marathons to benefit from exercise—a simple daily walk will do for most of us. But you'll be amazed at how much better regular exercise and healthy lifestyle habits can make you feel and how easy they are to practice once you get used to them.

Remember that your prevention plan includes a healthy, high-fiber diet, regular exercise, moderation, and rest and relaxation. We've already discussed diet, and I'll give you more practical tips on good eating in the coming chapters. This chapter deals with healthful exercise and lifestyle habits.

The first step to health and longevity is to pick healthy, long-living parents. However, since most of us did not have the foresight to do that, we must go to the second step and overcompensate by living a preventive lifestyle. Some of us are born with a tendency to develop high blood pressure, heart disease, diabetes, cancer, and other diseases. This tendency is written into our genes inherited from our parents, and we can't change it. Our exercise and lifestyle habits are things we can change. And, like diet, these habits also affect our risk for chronic diseases. It's never too late to change habits, and the sooner the better—for your current and your future health and happiness.

Why Exercise?

What would you pay for a newly discovered drug that could help you control your weight, build your strength and flexibility, tone your muscles, strengthen your heart and lungs, lower your cholesterol, control your blood pressure, reduce your risk and symptoms of disease, relieve stress and tension, elevate your mood, improve your sleep, increase your energy level, and help you live longer? For the cost of a good pair of walking shoes and a modest time investment, all these benefits can be yours.

Regular exercise offers tremendous physical and psychological benefits. You will be amazed at how much better you can feel by spending only two to three hours per week exercising. Even people in their eighties who have started a mild exercise program report big gains in energy, strength, and agility that they thought impossible at their age.

Regular exercise complements all the benefits of our prevention eating plan, but it cannot substitute for healthful eating. Marathon runners who load up on high-fat foods occasionally drop dead from fat-clogged blood vessels. While exercise can't compensate for bad eating, it does many wonderful things when combined with good eating.

Regular exercise gives those of us battling to lose or maintain weight a powerful new weapon. Remember that losing weight boils down to a simple equation between calories in and calories out. Watching what you eat works on the calories in side of the equation, while exercise works on the calories out side of the equation, producing a greater calorie deficit and faster weight loss.

Brisk walking burns about 100 calories per mile for the average person. Walking twelve miles weekly would result in a yearly loss of eighteen pounds with no changes in diet. If you improved your eating pattern at the same time, you could easily double or triple this loss without ever going on a diet.

Muscle tissue, not fat, is where most of our calories are burned. Exercise has an added advantage in that it helps build muscle, which in turn helps burn extra calories long after exercising stops. Studies have shown that continued regular exercise is one of the variables most strongly associated with permanent weight maintenance.

Contrary to what you might think, exercising does not usually make you more hungry. Rather, exercise helps us better regulate our appetite and balance our food intake more closely to actual calorie needs.

Beyond weight control, exercise offers several other important advantages. Exercise builds strength, muscle tone, endurance, and flexibility. All these attributes make our other daily chores easier, giving us more energy left over for things we enjoy.

Exercise strengthens the heart and improves circulation, lessening stress on vital body organs. In fact, inactivity is a risk factor for heart disease and a predictor of death from heart disease in healthy men. Exercise lowers blood cholesterol levels and levels of the artery-clogging LDL cholesterol. Exercise raises levels of the protective HDL cholesterol. Exercise lowers blood pressure and blood sugar and is useful in prevention and treatment of many diseases.

Exercise adds years to life *and* improves the quality of life. Studies of Harvard graduates show that men who burned more than 2,000 calories per week in exercise, equivalent to walking fifteen to twenty miles per week, had 25 to 33 percent lower death rates than men who did not exercise. With a calculator you can compute that every mile you walk adds an hour to your life. Our mathematically inclined son figured if you walked twenty-four miles per day you would live forever! However, I shared with Steve that the benefits of exercise for increasing longevity, for some unknown reason, decrease when you excede thirty-five miles per week.

Another recent study published in the *Journal of the American Medical Association* showed that people who were inactive had almost three times the death rate over an eight-year period than people who walked thirty minutes daily.

Besides physical benefits, exercise also helps us psychologically. Regular exercise causes our body to release chemical compounds called endorphins, which are natural mood elevators. Exercise is great for relieving stress and tension and is mentally relaxing. We sleep better and feel more energetic when we exercise regularly. Add these benefits to a toned, fit body and we can't help but feel better about ourselves when we exercise.

EXERCISE BENEFITS:
- Reduces risk for heart attack
- Decreases risk for developing diabetes
- Assists in weight management
- Decreases blood pressure
- Contributes to peaceful living
- Prolongs life and improves quality of life

The Good, Better, Best Exercise Plan

No matter what your age or current level of physical activity, you can begin an exercise program. It takes four to six weeks to reap the full benefits of regular exercise, so give it a try for at least this long. If you can keep going this long, you'll probably be hooked for life.

Regular exercise doesn't have to be hard, complicated, or excessive to be beneficial. In fact, studies show that walking thirty minutes a day reduces death rates almost as much as running twelve to sixteen miles weekly.

Our exercise plan has three levels—good, better, and best—depending on your level of health and the time you have available to exercise. A *good* exercise level corresponds to walking the equivalent of *twelve miles weekly*. It's best to spread the twelve miles out over three to five days to get maximal benefit. Level one is a minimal level of exercise we recommend for everyone. If you haven't exercised for a long time, you'll probably need to build up to this level very gradually. Just begin walking at a speed and distance you are comfortable with—even if it is only a slow stroll to the end of the block and back—and then gradually increase your intensity and distance as walking becomes easier.

A *better* exercise level corresponds to walking *twenty miles per week*. We recommend that people with diabetes, high blood pressure, or high blood cholesterol levels target this level after building up their distance and pace gradually.

The *best* exercise level corresponds to walking or slow jogging *thirty to thirty-five miles weekly*. We recommend this intensive level of exercise especially for people trying to lose weight or maintain their weight loss. While exercising at this level might seem like a big time commitment, it takes less time and effort and certainly less money than repeated enrollment in diet programs. If you choose to slow jog, you'll also be able to cover the distance a bit faster.

I like to recommend walking for exercise because it can be done almost anywhere by almost everyone. It also requires very little special equipment or extra driving or preparation time. With walking, traveling is no excuse for not exercising, since you can even walk hotel halls and stairs if necessary. Walking is also low impact and puts less stress on joints and tendons than other forms of exercise. Running shoes are your feet's best friends if you walk more than two miles at a time; go to a running shop and get shoes tailored to the needs of your feet.

Many people, however, also enjoy other forms of exercise or like to build variety into their exercise routine. If you prefer to swim, cross-country ski, bike, row, or do other forms of exercise, we have listed the equivalent of one mile of walking for several different activities. Simply multiply this amount by 12, 20, or 35 to determine how long to exercise at the good, better, and best levels.

WALKING EQUIVALENTS OF OTHER FORMS OF EXERCISE	
Activity	**Time or distance equivalent to walking 1 mile**
Jogging	1 mile
Biking	3 miles
Swimming	10 minutes
Rowing machine	12 minutes
Stationary bike	12 minutes
Aerobics	20 minutes
Active tennis	20 minutes
Active racquetball	20 minutes

Exercising Safely and Enjoyably

If you are over thirty-five years of age or have diabetes or a history of heart problems, consult your doctor before beginning an exercise program. If you are under thirty-five years of age and feeling well, you can begin your exercise program slowly and gradually increase the time and intensity. If you build up your distance and speed very gradually, perhaps over a few months, you'll be surprised at how effortless and painless it is to get in good shape.

Listen to your body when you are exercising—if it hurts or if you are stiff or sore the next day, you are probably doing too much too fast. Don't believe the addage "No pain, no gain." If you experience faintness, shortness of breath, unusually rapid heart beat, chest pain, dizziness, or blurry vision, stop exercising immediately and consult your doctor.

All the exercises we listed as options in our plan are aerobic—that is, they use oxygen while repetitively working the large muscles of the arms and legs. Anaerobic exercises like weight and nautilus training build muscle but may not offer as many health benefits as aerobic exercise. A weight lifting program does improve flexibility and complements an aerobic walking program.

When you exercise aerobically, you should be breathing a little heavily but not so you couldn't carry on a conversation. Experts tell us that our heart rate should be between 60 and 85 percent of our maximal heart rate when we exercise. You can determine your maximal heart rate by subtracting your age from 220. Then multiply that number by 0.6 and 0.85 to find out how many beats per minute your heart should be pumping when you exercise.

OPTIMAL HEART RATES DURING EXERCISE			
Age	**Suggested heart rate during exercise***	**Age**	**Suggested heart rate during exercise***
20	120 to 170	55	99 to 140
25	117 to 166	60	96 to 136
30	114 to 162	65	93 to 132
35	111 to 157	70	90 to 128
40	108 to 153	75	87 to 123
45	105 to 149	80	84 to 119
50	102 to 145		

*Beats per minute, 60 to 85 percent of maximum heart rate

Begin each exercise session with a brief warm-up and end each session with a brief cool-down. Warming up is a way of letting your body know that more vigorous exercise is coming. Warming up gets the blood flowing to large muscle groups and increases heart rate gradually. It also stretches the muscles to prepare them for exercise and to help prevent injury.

Cooling down slows the system down gradually after exercise, much like you turn down the throttle on a lawn mower before you shut it off. If we quit exercising abruptly when blood is still pouring out into the large muscles of the legs and arms, blood pools in these muscles and can cause faintness or dizziness. Lactic acid, a by-product of exercising, also builds up in these muscles and can cause stiffness and soreness the next day.

The length of time each individual needs to warm up and cool down varies. For most of us, five to ten minutes is adequate. Warm-up and cool-down can consist of some simple stretches to loosen up the muscles we are going to use. Hold the stretch instead of bouncing, and stretch just far enough to feel it but not so far that it hurts. If you are walking or jogging, you may also want to warm up with a slower pace and gradually pick up speed.

Regular exercise is fun once you get in the routine, and you have lots of different activities to chose from. Choose a form of exercise that you enjoy and that you can work most easily into your schedule. You need to plan time into your schedule for exercise, just as you set aside time to watch the news, read the newspaper, or do the dishes. If you want to arrange to exercise with someone else, that's fine. Just don't let the other person's failure to exercise be an excuse for you to quit too.

Making the Most of Daily Activities

Besides setting aside time for regular aerobic exercise, use every opportunity you can to build more activity into your daily routine. Park your car farther from work or from the shopping mall and walk a little farther. Better yet, walk or bike to work if you can. Walk your child to school or special activities instead of driving, helping your child develop good living habits while helping yourself.

Take stretching or walking breaks instead of coffee breaks at work, and use the stairs instead of the elevator whenever possible. Mow your lawn with a push mower instead of a riding one, and rake your own lawn instead of hiring it done.

Plan for active family vacations with opportunities for swimming, hiking, or touring on foot. Also, try to develop activities and hobbies. While bowling, gardening, car repair, woodworking, or golf aren't aerobic activities, they do require movement, and every little bit helps.

Moderation

Recently Jack Dudley was named America's Most Overworked Person. This sixty-one-year-old executive with a heart problem works fifteen-hour days and commutes a total of four hours per day. He says that he knows it is time to change, but he doesn't know how. "Isn't that awful?" he said.

Many people like Jack are in a rat race, and the rats are winning. Our prevention plan includes moderation as a critical element. Moderation includes not smoking, using moderation in alcohol and caffeine use, avoiding habit-forming drugs, and working in moderation. Medical authorities agree that avoidance of alcoholic beverages is healthier than consumption in moderation. But if you drink alcohol, limit yourself to seven drinks per week and don't exceed three in one day.

Most people should limit their caffeine intake to four cups of coffee or its equivalent in soft drinks per day. Some individuals have a chronic anxiety disorder and need tranquilizers and sleeping pills to function adequately. However, most people use these pills to burn the candle at both ends. They drink coffee to keep them alert and then use pills or alcohol to crash at night. All tranquilizers, sleeping pills, and antidepressants dull your mind and decrease your mental function. If you, like me, need all the brain power available to do your job, you, like me, should avoid these pills like the plague. Our rest and relaxation plan will help you relax and get your rest.

Rest and Relaxation (R & R)

Jack Dudley doesn't have much time for R & R either. The prevention plan teaches you to get adequate rest at night, take personal time each weekend, take a long weekend every three months, and take at least one week of relaxing vacation each year. But, you say, I don't have time to do that. Neither do I, but I do it—my doctor tells me I need to do it.

Let's start with sleep. Different people require different amounts of sleep, but most people require about seven hours per night. You can get by on less sleep, but you pay a price. If you run a chronic sleep deficit, you have no reserve and are more vulnerable to infections and life stresses. If you have less energy on Friday morning than you do on Monday morning, you probably are getting less sleep than you need. If you tend to sleep excessively during holidays, this also may indicate that you are accumulating a sleep deficit.

Because most of us overdraw on our sleep account during the week, we need to restore the balance on the weekend. If you are short on sleep, we recommend that you sleep late or take a two-hour nap on Saturday or Sunday. Even if you can't sleep, commit two hours of personal time to reading in bed or a comfortable chair to get some extra R & R.

Even if you get adequate rest, you need a break from your routine each quarter. We recommend a three-day weekend for R & R every three months. This should be a change of pace like visiting a nearby resort or some fun place to take your mind off your day-to-day world.

Finally, I feel that one week of restful vacation each year is essential for good mental health.

JIM'S DIARY: Before you ask, I'm going to tell you that I practice what I preach in the R & R arena. I lead a busy life as a doctor, researcher, teacher, lecturer, writer, husband, father, grandfather, Sunday school teacher, college trustee, and walker. To function well, I need about seven hours sleep a night. I can get by with less but I pay a penalty in decreased efficiency.

Because my schedule doesn't always afford the luxury of seven hours of sleep, I regularly take a nice nap on Sunday afternoons. I'm grouchy if I don't get my nap because I know that I need it. Each Wednesday night I spend two hours with my older granddaughter. On our date we shop, walk, and have frozen yogurt. My wife, Gay, and I go out to dinner every Friday evening and enjoy a relaxing evening of shopping or a movie.

Every November and February we get away for a three-day weekend. Last November we went to New York City to see Broadway plays, shop, and sleep late; the year before we went to Disney World. In February we often go to a nearby resort for three days of relaxation and good (healthful?) eating. Finally, each July we go to Hilton Head with our family for a week. I walk five or six miles before breakfast and two miles after dinner. We enjoy a family breakfast and frequently have dinner in a restaurant. This R & R pattern works for me and for many of my patients who try it and like it.

Pacing Your Life

But, you say, your entire day is booked solid and you barely have time to brush your teeth much less exercise? We all feel this way some time or another—it's an unfortunate symptom of our increasingly time-squeezed society. We have to juggle business meetings, work deadlines, little league baseball games, family get-togethers, housework, meal preparation, money management, commuting, church activities, and more. We're supposed to be a dedicated employee, loving spouse, doting parent, good citizen, and still have a little time left over for personal growth—a near impossible feat for most of us.

All these pressures cause stress, and stress has definite physical consequences that can compromise our health. Stress triggers an outpouring of adrenaline, a hormone that used to prepare humans for "fight or flight" in the olden days of saber-tooth tigers and wooly mammoths. If this built-up energy is not released, stress can contribute to problems like ulcers, headaches, stomachaches, bowel problems, asthma, arthritis, sleep disturbances, and sexual dysfunction. Though the role of stress in heart disease is still unclear, certain emotions like anger and hostility are strongly linked to heart disease risk.

We can define stress as a mental and physical reaction to external events. Stress is not all bad—life would be boring without a little stress. Most of us need to be comfortably challenged and motivated. Sometimes we even do our best work under stress. Stress also builds character and gives us resilience.

But too much or continual stress can wear us down and eventually cause burn-out. Physical signs of excessive stress include clammy hands, clenched jaws, flushing of the face, crying easily, difficulty sleeping, change in appetite, short temper, tense muscles, lack of motivation, and loss of interest in friends, family members, or social activities. Major life events like marriage, divorce, or death of someone close to us certainly cause stress. But it's often the smaller day-to-day stresses that wear on us the most.

Like everyone, you have your own threshold for tolerating stress and your own method for coping with it. If you're over your comfort threshold or if you don't have a spare minute for exercise, take a moment to think about your life stresses and pace.

List the main sources of stress in your life. These might be major stresses such as trauma and grief over the loss of a loved one, or minor but continually irritating stresses such as an overbearing boss or a constantly messy house.

Next, brainstorm on ways to deal with these stresses. You have three kinds of choices for each source of stress: you can do something to change or remove the source of stress; you can change the way you perceive and react to the source of stress; or, if you can't do either of these, you can find a good outlet to relieve your feelings of stress.

Maybe you can remove some of your sources of stress and pace your life more comfortably. If you have unresolved conflict in your life, or a situation you are not dealing with so well, confront it and get help if you need to. If a constantly messy house bothers you, hire a cleaning person. If you run from one meeting to the next all day and all evening, weed out some of the less important commitments.

If you are continually feeling rushed, maybe you need to plan your daily goals more realistically. You will probably accomplish just as much without the stress of thinking you should do more. Think about your goals and priorities in life. Preplan and schedule time for what's important, and learn to say no to the rest. Planning in time for health maintenance will save you time in the long run, much like regular car tune-ups and oil changes prevent time-consuming breakdowns in the future.

If you cannot change the source of stress, maybe you can change how you perceive the situation. Who really cares if your house is messy? Is it really that important? If you are stuck in a traffic jam that will make you late for a meeting, do you fidget and fret or relax and enjoy a few minutes of music? Try to turn the negatives into positives, look at obstacles as opportunities for growth and change, and smell the roses whenever you can.

Even with a positive thinking and action plan, dealing with a certain amount of stress is still inevitable. You need to find effective ways to release built-up stress and tension. Regular exercise is one of the best ways I know of to diffuse stress. Exercise releases built-up muscle tension and is mentally relaxing. When you feel like slamming your fist through the wall, take a walk or slam a tennis ball with your racket instead. And, you'll be doing yourself a big favor by choosing exercise as a stress reducer. Return to the list of exercise benefits earlier in this chapter to see what else you'll be getting along with reduced stress.

If you notice that your forehead is wrinkled, that your shoulders are raised and tense, or that your teeth hurt because you are clenching your jaw, take a few minutes to shut your eyes and concentrate on relaxing every muscle in your body, and then think of something pleasant. Some people recall a scripture verse or pray a short prayer to relax. Express your feelings instead of bottling them up—talk to someone if you can, or write your feelings down.

Take care of yourself by getting enough sleep and planning enough time to relax. Follow our R & R plan for six weeks and you'll find that taking time for relaxation and rejuvenation will substantially increase your ability to deal with the stressful situations in your life. Set aside enough time for hobbies, social activities, and personal growth. Without pre-planning and goal setting, these things often get squeezed out of our busy schedules.

Cigarettes and Other Harmful Substances

SUCCESS STORY:
John corrects an alcohol abuse problem.

John, a fifty-six-year-old real estate agent, came to see me about his high blood triglycerides. He also had high blood pressure requiring daily medication. During my routine history John told me that he consumed at least three to four alcoholic drinks per day; he probably drank more. Over the past five years, as business got more competitive, he'd doubled his alcohol consumption. He also had noted more irritability (quickly confirmed by his wife) and less energy and reported that he had more difficulty getting started in the morning.

John was concerned about his health, his blood pressure, and his triglycerides. At his first visit I alerted him that his excess alcohol intake was contributing to his health problems. He felt strongly that he was a "social drinker" and wanted to focus on diet and exercise. Our dietitian instructed him in our high-fiber prevention diet and we encouraged him to start walking two miles per day.

John adopted the diet and exercise program wholeheartedly and his triglycerides decreased into the normal range. With my coaxing he decreased his alcohol intake to three drinks per day. As he began to feel better he dropped the noon drink. After one year, he weened himself to one glass of wine in the evening. Gradually he changed to enjoying one or two glasses of wine at restaurants and stopped drinking at home.

With the reduction in alcohol intake, John noted he had more energy, felt good in the morning, and was more easygoing. His family testified to the improved family relationships. With the reduction in alcohol intake, the high-fiber diet, and walking twenty miles per week, John was able to stop using the blood pressure medicine. His triglycerides and blood pressure were normal and John was trimmer by twenty pounds after eighteen months on our prevention plan.

Cigarettes, alcohol, sleeping pills, tranquilizers, or other drugs are not good ways to cope with stress but are unfortunately outlets that many people turn to. These harmful substances might give temporary relief from stress but are likely to cause much more of their own stress in the long run.

The problem with quick fixes is that they do not get at the underlying causes of stress; they only cover them up. Alcohol depresses the central nervous system and impairs judgment. Drugs also impair judgment, damage the central nervous system, and many are illegal. Tranquilizers and sleeping pills are depressants and can be very addictive.

Cigarette smoking is the most widespread addiction in the world, and nicotine is as physically and psychologically addicting as cocaine or heroine. Cigarette smoking accounts for about 30 percent of deaths from heart disease, 30 percent of deaths from all cancers, and 80 to 85 percent of deaths from lung cancer.

The more you smoke, the greater your health risks. Every cigarette counts. People who smoke only half a pack of cigarettes daily have twice the risk of heart attack, three times the risk of stroke, two to four times the risk of sudden cardiac death, seven to twelve times the risk of lung cancer, and fifteen times the risk of chronic lung diseases as nonsmokers. Risks multiply even more if you also have high blood pressure or high blood cholesterol levels. It's no wonder a U.S. government report calls smoking the "largest preventable cause of death in America."

Smokers aren't the only ones affected by cigarette smoke. Spouses of heavy smokers experience two to three times more lung cancer than people living in smoke-free environments. Babies born to smoking mothers suffer more complications, birth defects, and low birth weights than babies of nonsmoking mothers. Children exposed to smoke in the home get more coughs, colds, and ear infections than children of nonsmokers.

How to Quit Smoking

If you smoke, chances are that you would like to quit or have tried quitting. Studies show that over 90 percent of people who smoke cigarettes would like to quit. Unfortunately, 60 to 70 percent of those who quit smoking start again within a few months.

It takes several tries for many people to quit smoking, but keep trying and you'll succeed. The benefits are well worth it. Your risk for heart disease starts dropping the minute you stop smoking. Heart disease risk is about one-half that of a nonsmoker one to two years after quitting and the same as a nonsmoker ten years after quitting.

About 80 percent of people who quit smoking experience symptoms of nicotine withdrawal such as irritability, headaches, sleep disturbances, and restlessness. These physical symptoms are strongest the first few days of quitting but can last a few weeks. Psychological craving for cigarettes can last a year or more.

Some people find that nicotine patches or nicotine chewing gum help them stop smoking when combined with behavior change and exercise. Both of these aids are available only by prescription, so discuss them with your doctor. Nicotine patches and gum help relieve symptoms of physiological addiction to nicotine but do not relieve psychological addiction.

About 70 percent of people who quit smoking gain a little weight, with the average gain being five pounds. Following our prevention plan, however, will help you control your weight. Even if you do gain a little, smoking is far more dangerous to your health than a few temporary pounds.

Most people who quit smoking do so on their own, but you don't have to do it alone. Your doctor, family, and friends can advise, encourage, and support you as you quit. The American Lung Association, the American Cancer Society, the National Cancer Institute, and the American Heart Association have several helpful pamphlets and programs for people trying to quit smoking. Local affiliates of these organizations as well as local clinics may also offer stop-smoking classes.

There is no one right way to stop smoking. Some people like to quit cold turkey, others like to cut back gradually. Most of all, you have to want to quit smoking and believe you can do it.

Think of why you want to quit and list the reasons. If you can't quit for yourself, do it for your spouse or children. Remind yourself of these reasons daily or any time you have a strong craving for a cigarette. Think of why you smoke and substitute another activity that serves a similar purpose.

Do you smoke to get a lift? Then go out and exercise for a lift. If you don't have time for a full-fledged aerobic work-out, walk a flight of stairs or do some stretches. Chewing gum or taking a cold shower may also help. Do you smoke to relax? Try deep breathing, reading a book, or taking a ten-minute catnap. Do you smoke because you are angry or tense? Try talking to someone or counting to ten instead of lighting up, or use vigorous exercise to help relieve tension. Do you smoke because you like fingering something? Then finger a pencil, paper clip, or coin instead.

Make it hard for yourself to smoke. Don't buy cigarettes or bring them in the house. If you are cutting down gradually, put your cigarettes in the back of the top closet shelf and twist two rubber bands around them. Treat yourself to a special reward for not smoking. Think of all the money and time you are saving.

Most of all, don't be discouraged if you slip off your plan; most people do at some time or another. Just because you have a few cigarettes after you've decided to quit doesn't mean you've failed. Remind yourself of why you want to quit and of all the positive steps you've taken toward quitting, then start again.

Tips to Stop Smoking

- Get your teeth cleaned and then brush them every time you want to smoke.
- Try making it one hour without a cigarette, then gradually lengthen the time.
- Smoke standing up. You'll be more aware of what you are doing.
- Smoke with your other hand. Smoking will seem more awkward.
- Change to a brand of cigarettes you don't like.
- Spend the money you would have used to buy cigarettes on a reward for yourself.
- Call a friend when you feel like smoking.
- Buy only one package of cigarettes at a time.

- Chew gum or snack on raw fruits and vegetables instead of smoking.
- If you are cutting down, don't empty your ashtrays.
- If you are quitting cold turkey, throw away all your ashtrays, matches, and lighters.
- Avoid coffee, alcohol, and other beverages you associate with smoking.
- Think of yourself as a nonsmoker.
- Quit smoking with a friend.
- Have your house and clothes cleaned to rid them of the smoky smell.
- If you slip off your plan, remind yourself of all the positive things you've done.

Making the Changes

Changing your lifestyle is a four-step process. First, you recognize the need to make changes. Second, you say "I can do that!" Third, you tailor the changes to your own living patterns. Fourth, you sustain the behavior long-term.

You have taken the first step by reading this book. Next you will say "I can do that!" for these important behaviors: 1) high-fiber, low-fat eating; 2) walking at least twelve miles per week; 3) using moderation by not smoking, limiting alcohol intake, avoiding sleeping pills and tranquilizers, and working a sensible schedule; and 4) endorsing the R & R practices of adequate sleep, weekend naps, quarterly long weekends, and yearly vacations.

Third, you will set realistic goals. If you only walk three or four miles per week you should not expect to walk thirty miles next week. We recommend the "50 percent guideline" and the "six-mile guideline" for increasing walking. If you walk eight miles this week, increase that by 50 percent and walk twelve miles next week by following the "50 percent guideline." If you walk twenty miles per week, increase that by six miles and walk twenty-six miles next week by following the "six-mile" guideline. Don't increase your activity by more than 50 percent or six miles, whichever is smaller, for next week. For most persons, these are realistic goals.

Fourth, you will make a commitment to sustain the activity. This needs to be a written commitment you can share with a family member or friend. Every six months you will need a checkup to see how your blood cholesterol, blood pressure, or weight is doing. You can do this at your doctor's office, at the nurse at work, or at your pharmacy.

In the back of part 1 of this book are two "I can do that!" worksheets. Fill one out, have someone who cares about your health witness it, and keep it. Fill the other out and return it to the HCF Nutrition Foundation and we will send you a newsletter every three months to help you sustain the High-Fiber Fitness Plan. Send in your worksheet and enhance your commitment to maintain these behaviors.

Chapter Action Plan

Goals

EXERCISE:

- *Good*—walk twelve miles per week
- *Better*—walk twenty miles per week
- *Best*—log thirty to thirty-five miles per week

MODERATION:

- Avoid tobacco, sleeping pills and tranquilizers
- If you use alcohol, drink less than seven drinks per week
- Avoid "workaholic" behaviors such as working excessive hours

REST AND RELAXATION:

- Get adequate sleep (at least seven hours per night)
- Spend two non-working hours weekly with family or friends
- Take a two-hour nap or two hours of personal time each weekend
- Enjoy one fun three-day break every three months
- Get away for one week of restful vacation each year

Prevention Note: Every mile you walk adds one hour to your life.

For More Help

The following organizations offer information to help you improve or maintain your level of healthfulness.

The American Lung Association
1740 Broadway
New York, New York 10019-4374
(212) 315-8700

National Cancer Institute
9000 Rockville Pike
Building 31, Room 4A-181
Bethesda, Maryland 20892
1-800-4-CANCER

The American Heart Association
National Center
7320 Greenville Avenue
Dallas, Texas 75231
(214) 750-5300

American Cancer Society
599 Clifton Road, N.E.
Atlanta, Georgia 30329
1-800-ACS-2345

5
COOKING MADE EASY

Recently Linda, a busy nursing supervisor, was in the supermarket. She studied a TV dinner carefully and then dropped it back in the freezer case saying, "No, I don't want to cook tonight." Linda, like 40 percent of Americans, doesn't like the way she eats but thinks it's too much work to change. Today's cooks, women and men, usually have fifteen minutes or less to get a meal on the table. They need recipes that are easy, quick, convenient, and tasty. People want to eat healthy but don't want to have to work hard at it.

Fortunately, good food doesn't have to be difficult to fix. Garden fresh vegetables and wholesome baked breads taste great by themselves and require little preparation. Fresh fruit travels anywhere and requires no preparation. A healthy salad of greens, vegetables, and small bits of meat or cheese takes just minutes to make. This chapter, along with the recipes, shopping tips, and menu plans elsewhere in this book, will help make healthful cooking easy.

Menu Magic

Although Americans eat away from home more and more these days, we still get about 70 percent of our calories from home-prepared foods. The kinds of foods we plan and cook at home, then, have a big impact on our health.

Everyone who eats does at least some menu planning, which simply means deciding what foods to eat together when. Menu planning can be meal to meal, day to day, or week to week, and it saves time, effort, and money. It also helps us plan for variety and wholesomeness.

Many busy people don't think they have time to plan meals ahead, but a few minutes of planning can save you hours of preparation weekly. It takes five to ten minutes for most people to plan out their meals for a week. How many times do you come home from work and spend five or ten minutes staring into the freezer trying to decide what to fix for dinner? After finally deciding, you discover you are missing some key ingredient and either have to run to the store or choose again.

When you plan meals ahead, you know what ingredients you need and can have them on hand, avoiding time-consuming trips to the grocery store and unnecessary purchases. You can defrost foods ahead so they are ready to cook when you get home. You can start recipes the night before for a mouth-watering dinner in minutes. You can cook and freeze double batches and get twice the mileage for half the effort. You can make better use of leftovers. You can assign your spouse or older child some cooking duties. You can even save your menu plans from week to week to use again.

Planning ahead also allows you to select nutritious foods on the run instead of succumbing to a barrage of handy garbage. Sometimes it seems easier to grab a handful of chips and a hot dog in a pinch when instead you could have grabbed a handful of blueberries and a sliced turkey sandwich if you had planned ahead.

Try taking five to ten minutes on the weekend to plan out your main meals for the week. Menu plans don't have to be elaborately detailed— just detailed enough to give you an idea of what foods to have on hand and what precooking steps you can take. If breakfasts and lunches are similar from day to day, you may just need to plan out your main dish and maybe a side dish or two for the evening meal. On days you know your schedule will be tight, you can plan a precooked meal or plan to go out.

Your menu plans don't have to be rigid either. If you've got some meal ideas down on paper, you may feel like fixing Wednesday's dinner on Monday. Or maybe something unexpected comes up and you use the precooked meal you planned for another night.

Since all of us are unique individuals, we all have unique eating styles. If you don't eat regular meals, then plan some of your mini-meals or snacks ahead of time. There's nothing wrong with grazing, just be sure what you're grazing on is good for you.

The whole family should be able to eat from the same menu plan. Individuals with lower calorie needs will take smaller portions, and individuals with greater calories needs will take larger portions. If you have children, there's no need to fix separate food for them. The American Academy of Pediatrics recommends a low-fat diet with plenty of grains, fruits, and vegetables for all children over two years of age. If your child is a fussy eater, try to plan at least one or two foods on the family menu each meal that you know your child likes. Toddlers and young children will also probably need additional snacks because of their limited stomach capacity, appetites, and attention spans.

When you plan your menus, remember to build your meals on high-fiber plant foods using the 1,2,3,4 plan of one serving of cereal, two servings of fruits, three servings of vegetables, and four servings of starches. Extend meats by combining them in main dishes with pasta, rice, grains, vegetables, or dried beans.

SMART FOOD CHOICES	
Choose:	Instead of:
Fresh fruits	Sweet desserts
Fresh vegetable salads	Gelatin or mayonnaise-based salads
Whole-grain rolls, muffins, or bagels	Doughnuts or sweet rolls
Popcorn or whole-grain crackers	Chips
Vegetable and broth-based soups	Creamed soups
Whole-grain breakfast cereals	Highly sugared cereals
Baked potatoes	French fries
Sliced turkey, ham, or chicken	Bologna or hot dogs
Skimmed broth, bouillon, or wine	Gravies, meat drippings, or high-fat sauces

Sometimes it seems easier to stick to old favorites, but trying a new recipe or food occasionally will expand your cooking repertoire. If you're looking for ideas, try including these foods in some of your meals:

BREAKFAST:
- Fresh fruits like cantaloupe, grapefruit, oranges, strawberries, bananas, or blueberries
- Buckwheat or oatmeal pancakes topped with applesauce or sweetened fruit
- Whole-grain breakfast cereals
- Whole-grain toast, English muffins, or bagels
- Plain yogurt with fresh fruit

LUNCH:
- Bean, pea, or vegetable soups
- Fresh vegetable salads topped with beans, lemon, or low-fat dressings
- Whole-grain crackers with low-fat cottage, mozzarella, or farmers cheese
- Sandwiches made with whole-wheat bread or pita pockets and sliced chicken, turkey, lean ham, or water-packed tuna
- English muffin topped with pizza sauce and mozzarella cheese
- Whole-grain French bread topped with ham, mustard, peppers, onions, and shredded low-fat cheese

SUPPER:
- Baked potato topped with low-fat cheese, nonfat sour cream substitute, or yogurt
- Squash or peppers stuffed with rice, pepper, onion, and lean beef
- Fresh vegetables sprinkled with lemon and herbs
- Casseroles with brown rice, bulgur, and dried beans
- Whole-wheat spaghetti with fresh tomato sauce and parmesan cheese
- Baked fish with lemon
- Baked salmon puffs
- Baked chicken with brown rice
- Stir-fry dishes with lots of vegetables mixed with beef, chicken, or pork
- Whole-grain rolls or French bread
- Tortillas filled with beans, lettuce, tomatoes, and nonfat yogurt

Use the handy menu planning grid at the end of this chapter to plan your menus for a week.

Quick and Simple Cooking Tips

You can cook great meals quickly and easily if you plan, choose the right foods, and have the right equipment. As you've already seen, a few minutes of menu planning will help you get meals on the table faster and with less effort.

Certain kitchen equipment and gadgets also simplify cooking. Buy a sturdy brush for cleaning vegetables and fruits, and throw away your peeler. A microwave is a must for any hurried kitchen. Microwaving food not only saves time but also saves more nutrients than traditional cooking methods. The time-bake feature on stoves is also handy for starting casseroles or baked dishes while you are away. If you time it right you can even set frozen dishes in the oven to thaw gradually and then start to cook before you come home, but you have to be careful not to leave thawed food sitting out more than a few hours.

Slow cookers are great for stewed meats, soups, chili, and beans. Just put the ingredients together before you go, set the temperature, and your meal is ready when you come home. Grilling is also a quick and tasty way to cook certain foods without messing up the kitchen or dirtying extra dishes. If you're lucky, you might even be able to get someone else to do it. Many people also find that food processors save precious preparation time.

The form in which you purchase foods can make food preparation easier. Today you can buy washed and cut vegetables, chopped onion and green pepper, ready-made salads, shredded cheese, and presliced and deboned meats. These items cost more but when you consider the cost of your time it may be worth paying for them.

Another alternative is to prepare your own convenience foods in batches as soon as you come home from the store. Cut vegetables up all at once instead of meal by meal and bag them individually. Shred a big block of cheese and freeze in portions used for cooking.

Another time-saving trick is to plan for leftovers. When you do cook, make double or triple batches and freeze ahead. Cooking large batches takes just minutes longer than single batches and gives you instant precooked meals for hectic days. If you brown ground beef or bake a chicken, brown or bake extra and freeze to use in soups or casseroles later.

When you plan meals, choose foods that cook fast or foods that cook slow but require little preparation. Fish, pasta, steamed vegetables, and stir-fry dishes cook quickly. Roasts, stews, and casseroles cook slowly but require little effort to assemble.

Here are some other tips for preparing certain foods:

VEGETABLES:
- Learn to enjoy the natural flavor of fresh vegetables by preparing them with little butter, salt, or dressings.
- Cook in a microwave when possible, saving both time and nutrients.
- Cook until just tender-crisp. They look and taste their best at this stage and retain more of their nutrients.
- Make your own dressings with lemon, vinegar, nonfat yogurt, or whipped low-fat cottage cheese.

BEANS:
- Use dried beans and peas in salads, as vegetable side dishes, and to replace meat in main dishes.
- Soak raw dried beans overnight to speed up cooking, or use canned beans processed without salt or fat.
- Try using a slow-cooker for bean soups, stews, and chilies.

FRUIT:
- Use fresh as a snack or dessert.
- Try the exotic and unusual such as kiwi, fresh pineapple, mangos, and berries for variety and interest.
- Leave peelings on whenever possible to increase fiber content and to simplify preparation.
- Use fresh to top yogurt, pancakes, and waffles.
- Use fresh and dried in muffins, pancakes, and quick breads.

GRAINS:
- Use whole-grain French bread, sourdough bread, or English muffins as a base for open-faced hot sandwiches or mini pizzas.

- Use fresh pasta for faster cooking.
- Mix chilled, cooked pasta with raw vegetables for salads.
- Use two egg whites in place of one whole egg in homemade baked goods.

DAIRY:
- Use skim milk in soups, puddings, baked products, and sauces.
- Substitute skim milk for evaporated milk in recipes.
- Use low-fat cottage cheese and substitute it for sour cream or mayonnaise whenever possible.

MEATS, POULTRY, AND FISH:
- Remove skin from chicken or turkey before cooking.
- Trim all visible fat before cooking.
- Grill, bake, broil, or boil rather than fry.
- Use nonstick vegetable oil spray if you do fry.
- Marinate tougher cuts of meat in vinegar, fruit juice, or wine mixtures overnight.
- Extend meat, poultry, and fish with grains, vegetables, or dried beans and peas in main dishes.
- Drain fat several times while cooking.
- Cook fish until just firm but still juicy.
- In a pinch, try cooking fish from the frozen state, doubling cooking time.

Menu Make-Over

Many small changes can add up to a huge difference in the nutritional value of your diet. Take a look at your own menus, and think of what changes you could make to improve them. Consider the following typical menu. For breakfast: pancakes, maple syrup, orange juice, and coffee; for lunch: pastrami sandwich with muenster cheese and Russian dressing on light rye bread, coleslaw, french fries, a pickle, and a soft drink; for supper: baked chicken, mashed potatoes with gravy, white dinner roll with margarine, and corn; for dessert: apple pie; and for a snack: corn chips.

How could you improve this menu? For breakfast, you could make buckwheat or other whole-grain pancakes and top them with applesauce or fresh blueberries instead of syrup for added fiber and nutrients. Likewise, replacing the orange juice with half a grapefruit would add extra fiber.

For lunch, you could shave calories and fat if you chose turkey with mustard and mozzarella cheese instead of pastrami. Add some lettuce and tomato in the sandwich to squeeze in more vegetables, and put it together with pumpernickel or whole-wheat bread for more fiber. Choose a fresh salad with light or diet dressing instead of the coleslaw made with mayonnaise, and choose milk instead of the soft drink.

For supper, take skin off the chicken before baking, and try baking in stewed tomatoes and onion or serving over a bed of brown rice. A baked potato topped with nonfat yogurt has more fiber and less fat than mashed potatoes smothered with gravy. So does a whole-wheat dinner roll with blackberry jam compared to the white dinner roll with margarine.

Try some fresh fruit such as sliced strawberries or peaches for dessert in place of the apple pie. For a snack, replace the corn chips with whole-wheat crackers, or consider a bowl of whole-grain cereal with milk.

Sensational Snacks

SUCCESS STORY:
Judy improves family snacking habits.

Judy has three sons, ages eight to thirteen, who eat everything that doesn't move at her house. She struggled to keep chips, crackers, and cookies on hand to feed them. Her boys indicated that they didn't like fruit and vegetables.

After Judy lost fifty pounds in our weight loss program she recognized that she could not maintain a healthy weight with all that junk food in her house. She began replacing cookies with tasty fruit such as bananas, apples, oranges, and tangerines. She bought pretzels instead of chips. She shopped for whole-grain, low-fat crackers and stocked low-fat cheese spreads. She also kept cut up vegetables in plastic containers. Instead of soft drinks she stocked vegetable and fruit juices. Within a few weeks her boys were enjoying their new snack foods and sharing them with friends who dropped in. Judy is doing well maintaining her weight with all of the high-fat temptations gone from the house.

Snacking is not wrong. In fact, snacking may even be healthier for you than eating just three square meals a day. Studies suggest that body metabolism rises after eating, so eating many small meals throughout the day may actually help you burn extra calories. Eating several times a day may also help lower blood cholesterol levels.

As for nutrition, it's not how you eat but what you eat that counts— so make your snacks good. You can't always plan your snacks, but you can plan to have the right snack foods around when you need them. Kids get a significant amount of their nourishment from snacks, so it's especially important for them to snack well. Below are just a few ideas.

GOOD-FOR-YOU SNACKS

Any kind of fresh fruit	Low-fat milk
Frozen bananas or grapes	Oat bran muffins
100 percent frozen fruit juice bar	Bread sticks
Whole-grain crackers	Half a sandwich
Bagels	Unsweetened cereal
Raisins	Whole-grain rolls
Nonfat yogurt	Leftovers
Raw vegetables	Plain popcorn
Rice cakes	Unsweetened applesauce
Toast with jam	Water-packed tuna
Low-fat cheese or cottage cheese	Sliced lean deli meats

Chapter Action Plan

Goals

MENU PLANNING

- Plan menus one week at a time.
- Make a weekly shopping list.

QUICK COOKING

- Stock staples commonly used.
- Use microwave, slow cooker, and time-bake option on oven to save time.
- Choose fast-cook meals for a short evening at home.
- Choose meals requiring minimal preparation when busy.

EFFICIENCY

- Shop once a week.
- Prepare double recipes and freeze half.
- Plan for leftovers to use later.

I Can Do That!

- Start by planning one or two meals more than you plan now. For example, if you never plan ahead, this Sunday plan one or two evening meals for the week. If you plan a few meals now, plan all your evening weekday meals this weekend. Use the planning grid that follows on the next page.
- Make a shopping list from your meal plan.
- The next time you fix your favorite casserole, make a double batch.

MENU PLANNING GRID

	Breakfast	Lunch	Supper	Snacks
Monday				
Tuesday				
Wednesday				
Thursday				
Friday				
Saturday				
Sunday				

6
SHOPPING MADE EASY

The typical supermarket has over twenty-six thousand foods on the shelves. No wonder we often feel overwhelmed by our grocery shopping task. Yet the foods you bring into the house largely determine what you and your family eat. If you buy a lot of soft drinks, potato chips, candy, sweet rolls, and ice cream, you and your family will eat a lot of these foods. If you buy a lot of oranges, melons, strawberries, carrots, broccoli, salad greens, beans, whole-wheat rolls, whole-grain cereals, rice, pasta, and lean meats, you and your family will eat a lot of these foods.

Planning your meals ahead, as discussed in the last chapter, greatly simplifies shopping. You can make a grocery list based on your menus, saving time and usually money. Shopping from a list also limits buying low-nutrition foods on impulse. Keep your grocery list taped to your refrigerator or cupboard door, and add to it as needed. As much as possible, organize your grocery list to match how foods are arranged in the store.

Try to shop for food less often, preferably about once a week. The average American shops for groceries 2.3 times per week, and people with small children shop even more frequently. Each time you go grocery shopping you use up valuable driving and store time. If you plan ahead and make a complete grocery list, you'll shop less often, and save more time. Investing in a freezer may also allow you to purchase extra foods and shop less often.

To speed up shopping, shop when the stores are less crowded. Right after work is usually the worst time to shop. Stores are usually congested just before supper, and you are also probably tired, hungry, and ready to buy anything that looks good. Shopping at a familiar store where you know the location of foods also saves time. Take turns shopping with your spouse or children if you can. Or you can hit the grocery store together and divvy up the list.

Stock up on nutritious staples each time you go to the supermarket. At the end of this chapter you'll find a list of basic, wholesome staples that should be a part of every healthy kitchen.

Flavor

In addition to stocking up on staples, you will want to have herbs and spices on hand to enhance the flavor of your new dishes. These should be kept in small glass jars away from heat and light. Many herbs and spices lose their zest after a year and may need to be replaced. We had some "collector's items" that were, maybe, ten years old. Replace your old herbs and spices and put the date on them so you will get their full benefit. The most common herbs that we use are: basil, bay leaf, dill, oregano, parsley, sage, tarragon, and thyme. The most common spices that we use are: cinnamon, cloves, cumin, curry, ginger, nutmeg, paprika, and pepper. The recipes in the back of the book will give you good ideas on which foods these herbs and spices enhance, and, with a little experimentation, you'll find others you like as well.

What to Buy and Why

Beans and Peas. Beans are naturally low in fat and provide more protein per penny than any other food; they are also great sources of both soluble and insoluble fiber. Choose any variety of dried beans or peas. Some of the more common beans include:

PINTO BEANS: Beige in color with streaks of brownish pink on the skin. Used in soups, South American and Mexican dishes.

NAVY BEANS: Dried white seed of the green bean used most often in soups and Boston baked beans.

RED KIDNEY BEANS: Curved dark red beans used most often in chili and red beans and rice.

LIMA BEANS: Fat, light-colored bean, native to Central America, eaten most often as a side dish or in soups and casseroles, particularly succotash.

BLACK BEANS: A staple food throughout South and Central America that is boiled, fried, spiced, and mixed with rice and other foods. Used in the traditional black bean soup.

CHICK PEAS: A nutty, light brown legume with a firm texture used in salads and to make humus, a seasoned paste (also called garbanzo beans).

LENTILS: Closely resembling split peas in both looks and use, lentils are a staple for people in underdeveloped countries throughout the world. Eaten most often as a side dish or in soups, stews, and casseroles.

Canned beans cook more quickly and are also a nutritious alternative to dried beans. They can be easily added to many soups, stews, and casseroles. Try to choose beans canned without added meat or fat, although even canned pork and beans contain less fat than many traditional main dishes.

Most canned beans contain 100 to 150 calories and 1 or less than 1 gram of fat per half-cup serving. Brands of canned beans in this range include:

- Bush's Baked Beans Seasoned with Bacon
- Bush's Deluxe Pork and Beans
- Bush's Vegetarian Beans
- Butter Kernel Chili Beans
- Green Giant Something Special Mexican Style Beans and Barbecue Beans
- Joan of Arc Chili Beans
- Trappey's Jalapeño Black-Eyed Peas
- Van Camp's Pork and Beans

Although "pork and beans" sounds much higher in fat and calories than vegetarian beans, the difference for many brands is minimal because such a small amount of pork is added. For example, Bush's Vegetarian Beans contain 110 calories and less than 1 gram of fat per serving, while Bush's Deluxe Pork and Beans contain 123 calories and 1 gram of fat per serving. You still need to check your bean labels, though. B & M Brick Oven Baked Beans contain 270 calories and 6 grams of fat per serving.

Beverages. Good beverage choices include skim milk, 100 percent fruit juices, vegetable juices, and good old water. If you want to get fancy, use unsweetened club soda, mineral water, or seltzer. Otherwise, nice cold water right out of the refrigerator will do just fine.

Regular sweetened soft drinks contain ten to thirteen teaspoons of sugar and 150 to 200 calories per twelve-ounce can. If you like soft drinks, choose diet drinks, but use them in moderation (two to three cans daily). Use decaffeinated coffees and teas in moderation also. Alcoholic beverages supply lots of calories void of vitamins or minerals and should also be limited to a maximum of seven drinks weekly.

Breads. Choose breads, buns, bagels, English muffins, and pita pockets with a whole grain (such as 100 percent whole-wheat flour—not just wheat flour) listed as the first ingredient whenever possible. When these choices are not available, enriched white breads are also good sources of complex carbohydrates, and they are low in fat. Wheat bran or oat bran muffins are also good sources of fiber and complex carbohydrates but can be laden with fat. Choose breads, rolls, and muffins with 2 grams or less of fat per serving.

Cereals. Like breads, cereals are a great source of complex carbohydrates and fiber. Choose cooked and ready-to-eat cereals with 3 grams or more of fiber, 5 grams or less of sugar, and 1 gram or less of fat per serving. Below is a partial listing of cereals that meet these guidelines. Examples include the following:

READY-TO-EAT:
- All Bran with Extra Fiber
- Fiber One
- Oat bran
- Shredded Wheat
- Shredded Wheat 'n' Bran
- Spoon Size Shredded Wheat
- Uncle Sam
- Whole Grain Total
- Whole Grain Wheat Chex
- Whole Grain Wheaties

COOKED:
- H-O Quick Oats
- Instant oatmeal
- Maypo
- Oat bran
- Old Fashioned Oats
- Quick Oats
- Wheatena

Crackers. Did you know that many crackers are fried? Ritz crackers, Rye Crisps, and many similar crackers are deep fried in oil and are high in fat. Look for crackers that contain less than two grams of fat per serving. Examples include:

- Nabisco Honey Graham and Graham
- Sunshine Krispy Original Saltines
- Soup, chowder, and oyster crackers
- Ak-Mak
- Wasa Heart Rye and Sesame Wheat Crispbread
- Kavli Whole Grain Crispbread
- Old London Melba Toast, wheat
- Master Old Country Hardtack

Dairy Products. If you're still using whole milk, cut down to low-fat milk. If you're using low-fat milk, cut down to skim milk. This doesn't sound like much of a change, but for every percent of milk fat you cut out per cup, you save 40 calories. If you drink two cups of milk daily, that's a calorie savings equivalent to eight pounds of body weight per year. Many companies are also now marketing lower-fat, reduced-calorie versions of popular cheeses:

- Kraft Light Naturals (mozzarella, Cheddar, Colby, and Monterey Jack)
- Kraft Healthy Favorites (Monterey Jack, mild Cheddar, and American)
- Kraft Free Singles (nonfat pasteurized processed cheese product)
- Healthy Choice Fat-Free Singles (nonfat pasteurized process cheese product)
- Borden Lite-Line (Swiss, Colby, and American)

Some cheeses are very high in fat and calories. Choose low-fat cheeses such as part-skim ricotta, part-skim mozzarella, string cheese, nonfat or low-fat cottage cheese, and reduced-calorie cheese. Substitute whipped nonfat cottage cheese or nonfat yogurt for sour cream. Choose nonfat, plain yogurts and add your own fresh fruit for flavor.

Eggs and Egg Substitutes. Since egg yolks contain large amounts of cholesterol, use egg substitutes such as Egg Beaters and Egg Scramblers when possible, or substitute two egg whites for one egg with yolk. When buying eggs, buy small or medium-sized eggs.

Fats and Oils. Buy nonstick vegetable oil sprays; monounsaturated oils such as canola (rapeseed) oil or olive oil; and polyunsaturated oils such as safflower, sunflower, and corn oil. As we discussed earlier, canola and olive oil are our main recommendations because they are rich in monounsaturated fats; try to avoid saturated fats and use moderation in polyunsaturated fats. Buy margarine in the tub with one of these liquid oils listed as the first ingredient, or try a diet margarine that has added water. Avoid hard stick margarines or solid vegetable shortenings with hydrogenated fats listed as the first ingredient—these are no better for you than butter. Also, beware of products with palm or coconut oil listed in the first few ingredients. If you have trouble giving up real butter, try a butter-margarine blend.

Choose diet or low-fat salad dressings with sixteen or fewer calories per tablespoon. Examples include:

- Kraft Free Thousand Island, Italian, and Blue Cheese
- Hidden Valley Ranch Take Heart Blue Cheese
- Hidden Valley Ranch Low-Fat Italian Parmesan
- Kraft Oil-Free Italian
- Wish-Bone Healthy Sensation Italian and Ranch
- Wish-Bone Lite Sweet 'N Spicy French
- Wish-Bone Lite Italian
- Newman's Own Light Italian

Try low-fat mayonnaise or, better yet, make your own mock mayonnaise with whipped nonfat cottage cheese.

Fish and Seafood. Although some fish contain more fat than others, almost all plain fish and seafood are good choices. In fact, the more fatty fish such as salmon, tuna, mackerel, sea trout, bluefish, herring, and anchovies contain more omega-3 fatty acids, which may help protect against heart disease.

Buy tuna and salmon packed in water instead of oil. Avoid prebreaded fish or seafood, which are also prefried and high in fat. Look for fresh fish and seafood that is firm, mild-smelling, and slightly translucent. Freeze fresh fish immediately or use it within one to two days. Frozen and locally caught fish are sometimes cheaper than fresh fish that has been flown in.

Frozen Dinners. Frozen dinners can save time and effort and still fit in with your prevention diet. Just look for the same things in buying a frozen dinner that you would look for in planning a homemade dinner, then round out the meal with whatever is missing.

Choose frozen dinners that emphasize plant foods—mixtures of meat (or other protein) and vegetables or meat and grains such as pasta or rice. If your dinner is frozen lasagna, toss up a quick salad with low-fat or diet dressing, add a whole-wheat roll or slice of bread, and a glass of skim milk. Frozen dinners with breaded meats are usually too high in fat. Salisbury steak, dinners with cheese sauce, and pot pies are also usually high in fat. Look for frozen dinners with less than 10 grams of fat (equivalent to about 30 percent of calories for a 300-calorie dinner) and 800 milligrams or less of sodium. Many lines of light and lean frozen dinners are available today, including:

- Stouffers Lean Cuisine
- Weight Watchers Low-Fat, Ultimate 200, and Smart Ones
- Healthy Choice
- The Budget Gourmet Light and Healthy
- Ultra Slim Fast
- Le Menu Healthy
- Banquet Healthy Balance

Choose frozen pizzas with a single layer of cheese topping or cheese and vegetables. You can also make your own quick pizza by using a prepared pizza crust, prepared pizza sauce, shredded part-skim mozzarella cheese, and fresh sliced vegetables.

Fruits. If you don't have the time to even peel a banana, buy cut-up fresh fruit at the salad bar in your supermarket. This makes a great appetizer, side dish, or dessert for your meal. Top with low-fat yogurt sweetened to taste with Equal, fat-free frozen yogurt, or brown sugar.

All fresh fruits are good fiber sources and should be nutritional staples in your diet. Citrus fruits, kiwi fruit, mangos, melons, papayas, strawberries, guava, and starfruit are good sources of vitamin C. Cantaloupe, apricots, nectarines, persimmons, and papaya are good sources of vitamin A. Keep a few apples, oranges, grapefruit, or other fruits that store well handy at all times, then supplement this supply with more perishable fruits after each shopping trip.

Try some less commonly eaten fruits such as fresh pineapple, blueberries, raspberries, starfruit, or kiwi occasionally for a special treat or dessert. Even though these fruits cost a little more, they are probably still less expensive than low-nutrition choices such as frozen desserts, packaged cakes, or snack mixes.

Although fresh fruits contain more fiber and nutrients than processed fruits, canned, frozen, and dried fruits are still good nutritional choices. When buying canned fruit, select fruit packed in its own juice with no added sugar. Choose real fruit juices containing 100 percent fruit juice rather than fruit drinks, which often contain only 10 to 15 percent real fruit juice and lots of added sugar. Buy frozen fruits packed plain or in their own juice rather than in sugared syrup. Dried fruits are especially good fiber sources but are also a more concentrated source of calories and may cause tooth decay. Use them sparingly.

Grains. All plain pastas, rice, and other grains are good choices and great sources of complex carbohydrates. Buy a lot of them, and eat them often.

Whenever you can, choose whole grains such as whole-wheat pasta, brown rice, oatmeal, cornmeal, bulgur, and barley for added fiber and nutrient content. Oat bran is also an excellent source of fiber, particularly of cholesterol-lowering soluble fiber.

Use packaged pasta and rice mixes cautiously. They usually contain high levels of sodium and fat when prepared according to package directions. When you make these mixes at home, skip or cut down on added fat. If you are concerned about sodium intake, add only part of the seasoning packet. Use lighter tomato-based sauces such as marinara over pasta rather than cream, cheese, or heavy meat sauces.

Meats. To get the leanest cuts, choose round, loin, sirloin, flank, and extra-lean ground beef. For pork, choose tenderloin, leg, shoulder, boiled ham, and Canadian bacon. For lamb, choose leg, arm, loin, and rib. Although organ meats such as liver, kidney, sweet breads, and heart are high in nutrients, they are also very high in cholesterol.

For poultry, choose turkey, chicken, and game hens. Be sure to remove the skin before cooking, or buy skinless chicken or turkey breasts. One-half of the calories in chicken are in the skin. As usual, any pre-breading of poultry at least doubles the fat and calorie content.

Most supermarkets now carry a good selection of lean deli meats. Buy sliced chicken breast, roast beef, roast turkey, or lean ham. The same choices also apply to packaged luncheon meats. As a general guide, select luncheon meats that are 95 percent or higher fat-free. Salami, pastrami, bologna, hotdogs, brats, and sausages have double or more the fat of these leaner meats. Even turkey hotdogs and the new leaner sausages offer only modest improvement over their regular counterparts.

Snack Foods. Of course, foods in most of the other categories make good snacks, especially fresh fruits and vegetables. As far as traditional snack foods go, however, good choices include plain popcorn (air-popped or microwave popcorn with 1 gram or less added fat per three-cup serving), pretzels, rice cakes, popcorn cakes, and no-oil tortilla chips. Although most cookies are high in fat and calories, better cookie choices include oatmeal cookies, arrowroot cookies, fig or other dried fruit bars, vanilla wafers, gingersnaps, and graham crackers. Diet gelatins and puddings are also alternative snack choices.

Soups. Creamy soups or soups in a gravy base are usually high in fat and calories. Cream of mushroom soup, for example, contains 131 calories, 11 grams of fat, and 0 grams of fiber compared to the 64 calories, 1 gram of fat, and 1 gram of fiber in vegetable soup. Choose broth-based soups such as minestrone, chicken noodle, chicken and rice, or vegetable soups, which emphasize pasta, rice, and vegetables. Canned soups can be high in sodium. If you need to limit your sodium, many lines of low-sodium soups are now available.

Vegetables. If preparing a salad for one or two, pick your choice greens, tomatoes, pepper strips, garbanzo beans, nuts, and other salad items at the supermarket salad bar. Rearrange in your own salad bowls for a nice change-of-pace. Also pick up some baby carrots for your lunch bag.

As are fruits, all fresh vegetables are good nutritional choices and are high in fiber (remember to leave the peeling on when preparing vegetables). Carrots, broccoli, sweet potatoes, winter squash, spinach, and other greens are good sources of vitamin A. Broccoli, tomatoes, spinach, green peppers, potatoes, Brussels sprouts, and cabbage are good sources of vitamin C. We recommend that you use fresh vegetables whenever possible for fiber and nutrient content. Canned and frozen vegetables, however, are good choices too. Some canned vegetables and vegetable juices can be high in sodium, although many low-sodium brands are now available. Keep packages of frozen vegetables handy in the freezer, but choose plain vegetables rather than those packed in higher-calorie cream or cheese sauces. Many grocery stores also sell prepared salads in the deli. Buy the green, leafy salads rather than mayonnaise-laden creamy-type salads.

Food Labels at a Glance

Following the National Nutrition Labeling and Education Act of 1990, a major effort by several government agencies has resulted in the most massive food label reform in America's history. These new labeling laws now require standard nutrition labels on virtually all foods. The new labels are designed to help consumers make the most healthful food choices.

Although reading labels might sound time-consuming, the new labels are streamlined, allowing you to gather a load of information at a glance. And once you've studied choices in a particular food category, you'll know what brand to buy in the future without having to compare labels.

Food packages provide three types of labeling information: ingredient labeling, nutrition labeling, and health claims. Under the new regulations, all food products, even those with standards of identity, must list ingredients in order by weight. The most prominent ingredient is listed first.

The nutrition labeling is now provided on a uniform panel called "Nutrition Facts." This panel gives information on the amount per serving of total calories, total fat, saturated fat, cholesterol, sodium, total carbohydrate, dietary fiber, sugars, protein, vitamin A, vitamin C, calcium, and iron. The panel also compares the quantity of these nutrients to a person's needs by listing "% Daily Value."

Nutrition Facts		
Serving Size ½cup (114g)		
Servings Per Container 4		
Amount Per Serving		
Calories 260	Calories from Fat 120	
		% Daily Value*
Total Fat 13g		**20%**
Saturated Fat 5g		**25%**
Cholesterol 30mg		**10%**
Sodium 660mg		**28%**
Total Carbohydrate 31g		**11%**
Dietary Fiber 0g		**0%**
Sugars 5g		
Protein 5g		
Vitamin A 4%	Vitamin C 2%	
Calcium 15%	Iron 4%	

* Percent Daily Values are based on a 2,000 calorie diet. Your daily values may be higher or lower depending on your calorie needs:

	Calories:	2,000	2,500
Total Fat	Less than	65g	80g
Sat Fat	Less than	20g	25g
Cholesterol	Less than	300mg	300mg
Sodium	Less than	2,400mg	2,400mg
Total Carbohydrate		300g	375g
Dietary Fiber		25g	30g

Calories per gram:
 Fat 9 • Carbohydrate 4 • Protein 4

The Daily Values are based on 2,000 calories, but, for the benefit of those with higher calorie needs, a footnote also gives values based on 2,500 calories. Daily values are set at 30 percent of calories from fat, 10 percent of calories from saturated fat, 60 percent of calories from carbohydrate, and 10 percent of calories from protein. For fiber, daily values are set at 25 grams of fiber for 2,000 calories and 30 grams of fiber for 2,500 calories.

For the first time, nutrition panels now also list calories from fat right next to total calories. To see what contribution fat makes to the product's total calories, simply divide calories from fat by total calories and multiply by 100. For example, in this product, 120 calories from fat divided by 260 total calories multiplied by 100 equals 46 percent of total calories from fat. While your total diet should contain less than 30 percent of calories from fat, this does not mean that any food with more than 30 percent of calories from fat is bad; it just has to be balanced with other lower-fat foods.

Up until recently, many food manufacturers made questionable health claims for their products. Terms like "light" or "reduced" were used very loosely, leading to unclear and sometimes deceptive advertising. Under the new labeling regulations, only certain health claims can be made on labels. These claims include the following relationships:

• Calcium and reduced risk of osteoporosis
• Fat and reduced risk of certain types of cancer
• Saturated fat and cholesterol and reduced risk of coronary heart disease
• Fiber-containing grain products, fruits, and vegetables and reduced risk of cancer
• Fruits and vegetables and grain products that contain fiber and reduced risk of coronary heart disease
• Sodium and reduced risk of hypertension (high blood pressure)

The new regulations also set standard and clear definitions for the following terms:

FREE: Contains either none or virtually none. Used for describing calories, fat, saturated fat, cholesterol, sodium, and sugars.

LOW: fat—3 grams or less per serving; saturated fat—1 gram or less; sodium—less than 140 milligrams; cholesterol—less than 20 milligrams; calorie—less than 40 calories.

LEAN and EXTRA LEAN: Used for meat, poultry, and seafood. Lean—less than 10 grams of fat, 4 grams of saturated fat, and 95 milligrams of cholesterol; extra lean—less than 5 grams of fat, 2 grams of saturated fat, and 95 milligrams of cholesterol.

HIGH: One serving contains 20 percent or more of the daily value.

GOOD SOURCE: One serving contains 10 to 19 percent of daily value.

REDUCED: A nutritionally altered product that contains 25 percent less of a nutrient or calories than the regular product.

LESS: A food, whether nutritionally altered or not, that contains 25 percent less of a nutrient or calories than another food.

LIGHT: A nutritionally altered food that contains one-third fewer calories or half the fat of the reference food, and half the sodium of the regular product.

MORE: Contains 10 percent more of the daily value of a nutrient than another food.

Chapter Action Plan

Goals

- Make a list and check it twice—you'll find out which foods are naughty or nice, and you'll save time.

- Pick these items:

Beans and peas. Have dried pinto or navy beans on hand for your slow cooker, dry lentils for soup, frozen peas for a side dish or salad, canned beans for chili, and a host of other main dishes and side dishes.

Beverages. Keep frozen fruit juices and canned vegetable juices on hand as well as your favorite mineral water.

Breads. Have bagels, English muffins, and whole-wheat bread in the freezer for quick meals and snacks.

Cereal. Stock your pantry with oatmeal, oat bran, wheat bran cereal, and Wheat Chex for cooking, muffins, and snacks.

Crackers. Buy whole-wheat, rye, and other low-fat crackers for snacks.

Dairy Products. Use skim milk, low-fat cheeses, nonfat sour cream, reduced-fat (Neufchâtel) cream cheese and nonfat yogurt and frozen yogurt.

Egg Products. Use egg substitutes or egg whites.

Fats and Oils. Buy canola oil for most cooking unless olive oil works best. Use liquid or tub margarines. Choose low-fat salad dressings.

Fish and Seafood. Keep water-packed tuna and canned salmon on hand, and have frozen fillets available for quick meals.

Frozen Dinners. Select low-fat entrees for quick meals.

Fruits. In addition to fresh seasonal fruit, keep canned and frozen berries, peaches, and other fruit for salads and desserts.

Grains. Keep quick cooking rice and barley on hand for quick meals.

Meat. Choose poultry and the leanest cuts of beef and pork. Have a supply of frozen ground turkey available for main dish casseroles and chili.

Pasta. Keep a variety of spaghetti, noodles, and other pastas in the cupboard for quick meals.

Snacks. Have pretzels, raisins, nonfat tortilla chips, salsa, popcorn, and other items available for the inevitable snacks.

Soups. Keep canned and dehydrated low-fat soups available for cooking and quick soups.

Vegetables. When you don't have time to peel, slice, dice, and chop, buy them already prepared at the supermarket. Also keep an assortment of canned and frozen vegetables on hand.

"Basics" Shopping List

- Brown rice
- Dried beans and peas
- Canned beans
- Canned salmon or tuna packed in water
- Canned fruits packed in juice
- Egg substitute
- Fresh fruits
- Fresh vegetables
- Frozen fish fillets
- Frozen vegetables
- Fruit juices
- Lean meats
- Low-calorie and diet dressings
- Low-fat cheeses
- Nonfat yogurt
- Oatmeal or oat bran
- Rice cakes
- Pasta
- Popcorn
- Skim milk
- Vegetable juices
- Whole-grain breads and rolls
- Whole-grain cereals
- Whole-grain crackers

I Can Do That!

• Choose two food categories from the above list in which you make some not-so-healthful choices. Review the related sections in this chapter and write down the choices you will make in the store next time.

(For example: *I Can Do That! Beverages—buy flavored mineral water instead of soda pop. Snacks—buy pretzels and nonfat tortilla chips instead of potato chips.*)

_____

_____

_____

_____

_____

_____

_____

7
EATING OUT
MADE EASY

A highlight of my week is meeting Gay for dinner on Fridays. You probably eat out frequently, as we do, for pleasure and practicality. Americans dine out an average of four times a week, eating 30 percent of all our meals away from home and 8 percent of all our meals in the car. We spend forty cents of every food dollar away from home including sixteen cents of each dollar at fast food restaurants.

While many diet plans tell you to avoid eating out, we'd like you to eat out as often as you want and to enjoy doing it. The same principles of the 1,2,3,4 plan apply to eating away from home. Select menu choices that emphasize plant foods—fruits, vegetables, grains, and legumes. Since Americans have become more health conscious, almost every restaurant has at least a few healthful choices available.

At a fast food restaurant you can choose a lean hamburger or sliced beef sandwich with a side salad. At a full-service restaurant you can load up on fresh bread or rolls, pasta or rice dishes, vegetable soup, or salad. You might also order a fresh fruit cup or an extra vegetable to complement your meal. At a vending machine you can choose plain yogurt, a piece of fruit, or pretzels.

And remember, it's your total diet balance over time that counts. If you eat out infrequently, an occasional splurge on a steak, Big Mac, or cheesecake won't shift your balance much. But the more often you eat out, the more care you'll need to take to choose carbohydrate- and fiber-rich plant foods.

When you eat out, practice a few critical skills. As always, *take a few minutes to preplan.* Do you often find yourself eating away from home on impulse because your errands took longer than expected or there's not time in between activities to go home and eat? If you think through your activities before you leave home, you might anticipate a time crunch and pack a sandwich or grab a piece of fruit to take along.

Or, when you make a conscious decision to eat out, think about where you'll go ahead of time. Where you eat greatly influences what foods you'll have to choose from and ultimately what goes into your stomach. You might decide to go to Arby's where you can get a lean roast beef sandwich instead of stopping at Kentucky Fried Chicken, for example. Or you might decide to go to a cafeteria where you can get fresh fruit, a salad, and a sandwich made to order. If you're not sure what's on the menu, you can call ahead and find out. When you know where you're going to eat out, you might even decide what you're going to order ahead of time.

Also, *learn to ask questions about how food is prepared.* Caution words include: breaded, fried, battered, creamed, stuffed, scalloped, au gratin, or served with sauce or gravy. If you're not sure how a food is prepared, ask.

Finally, *don't be shy about making special requests at restaurants.* You might ask that the fish be broiled without added fat, that the butter be left off the vegetables, or that dressings and sauces be served on the side. You can also ask if items not on the menu, such as fresh fruit or skim milk, are available. Some restaurants will prepare a vegetable plate for you even though it's not listed on the menu. With more and more people concerned about diet and health, most restaurants are used to special requests and will make every effort to accommodate reasonable requests.

Americans eat away from home in many different situations, among them a relaxing dinner at a full-service restaurant, a stop-and-go meal at a fast food restaurant, a quick bite at a deli, a brown bag lunch brought to work, a passing nibble at the mall, a missed lunch made up at a vending machine, an airline meal, or a cafeteria lunch. We'll give you healthful suggestions for each of these situations in the sections that follow.

Brown Bag Lunches

Brown bag lunches are home-prepared foods eaten out. And they don't have to be boring. You can use a variety of breads and fillings for sandwiches—a brown bag tradition. Or you can use yogurt, cottage cheese, and salads for variety. If hot foods appeal to you more, try soups, stews, and casseroles in a thermos to be heated later in a microwave.

Consider the typical sandwich lunch—some type of lean meat on two slices of whole-wheat bread with vegetable slices and a piece of fruit. This is a good basic bag lunch, but if you want greater variety, try varying the bread and filling you build your sandwich with and add some interesting extras. For example:

BREADS
- Rye or pumpernickel bread
- Oatmeal bread
- Whole-grain English muffin or bagel
- Whole-wheat French bread
- Pita pocket
- Sub roll
- Hamburger or hard bun
- Tortilla shell
- Crackers

FILLINGS
- Lean sliced beef, turkey, chicken, or ham
- Water-packed tuna or salmon moistened with cottage cheese
- Low-fat cheese
- Mashed, cooked dry beans

EXTRAS
- Lettuce or spinach leaves
- Alfalfa or bean sprouts
- Sliced onion, cucumber, or tomato
- Shredded carrots
- Crushed pineapple
- Sliced apples, pears, or bananas

If sandwiches don't appeal to you, try fresh salads, plain yogurt with fruit, crackers and vegetable slices with cottage cheese dip, or cold brown rice or pasta salads with bits of cooked meat and vegetables. Or, you can bring hot foods such as vegetable soup, baked beans, chili, casseroles, or leftovers in a thermos. Many work places now have refrigerators and micro-waves, making an almost endless variety of brown bag lunches possible. Whatever you choose to bring for lunch, round out the meal by including at least one fruit and one vegetable.

JIM'S DIARY: Gay, bless her heart, fixes me a sack lunch about four days a week. As you know, I'm a creature of habit and have a similar lunch each time. This includes twelve ounces of V-8 juice, two oat bran muffins, a sandwich bag filled with vegetables (broccoli, carrots, cauliflower, celery, and/or radishes), and fruit (apple, grapes, or an orange). I enjoy this and eat it at the faculty meeting where pizza or sandwiches are available. Sometimes I will have a cookie for dessert.

Traveling

Traveling doesn't automatically mean giving up healthful food. In fact, traveling healthy today is fairly easy if you take charge of your meals and use a little creativity. Much of our advice on eating in restaurants applies to traveling, but here are some extra things you can do to make healthful traveling even easier.

When you travel by air, request a special meal ahead of time. Most airlines offer about twenty different special meals for health or religious preferences at no extra charge, but you must request these meals eight hours or more ahead of time. When you call for your ticket, get in the habit of booking your meal while booking your flight and seats. Special airline meals usually include heart-healthy, light, vegetarian, low-cholesterol, low-sodium, and diabetic choices. These meals are often not only more nutritious but also more tasty than regular airline meals.

Order fruit or vegetable juice instead of soft drinks in the air, and look for alternatives to the traditional bag of peanuts. You might buy a piece of fresh fruit, some nonfat yogurt, or a pretzel in the airport to take with you on the airplane.

For hotel stays, consider bringing some nonperishable foods in your suitcase. Try canned fruit juice, small boxes of cereal, and packages of instant oatmeal for a quick and nutritious hotel breakfast. You can purchase a carton of milk the night before and keep it on ice until morning. Small packages of crackers, individual applesauce cartons, and whole fruit also travel well. You can even carry some plastic spoons and a small pocket-knife for cutting fruit.

For car trips, bring a small cooler with canned fruit and vegetable juices, fresh fruit and sliced vegetables, low-fat cheese, crackers, peanut butter, and dried fruit. You might think it takes a little extra time to pack these, but think how much time it takes to stop and find a place to eat. And if you stop at a scenic roadside rest area, you'll be more inclined to walk around and get a little exercise at the same time.

Vending Machines and Convenience Stores

More and more people today make their snacks and mini-meals from pre-pared foods in vending machines and convenience stores. The basic candy and soft drink machines now usually carry cracker or fruit juice alternatives. The larger machines carry sandwiches, single-serving canned foods, and a variety of snacks.

Good vending machine choices include turkey, chicken, or ham sand-wiches (you can decide whether or not to use the separate mayonnaise package), broth-based soups, plain yogurt, pretzels, animal crackers, and whole fruit or fruit juice. If sandwiches are not available, choose a ham-burger over a hot dog for higher nutrient and lower fat content.

Salad Bars

Fortunately, many restaurants—even fast food restaurants—now offer salad bars to complement their regular entrees. You can use salad bars as a main or side dish. But even though salad bars sound healthful, some choices are better than others.

Build your salad on fresh greens such as lettuce and spinach, then pile on the plain vegetables and beans. Frequent salad bar stars include peppers, mushrooms, carrots, broccoli, cauliflower, sprouts, onions, tomatoes, celery, garbanzo and kidney beans as well as fruits such as pineapple and raisins. Choose diet or low-calorie salad dressings. The average 100-calorie greens and vegetable salad can be overwhelmed by the 200 to 300 calories in the three to four tablespoons of high-fat salad dressing that many people use.

Top salads with bread crumbs, lean chopped ham, and chick peas or kidney beans. Many other salad toppings, such as shredded cheese, bacon bits, seeds, olives, and Chinese noodles, are high in fat and calories. You can often get your half-ounce of nuts here by taking a tablespoon of chopped nuts or about twelve pecan halves.

Three-bean salad, oil-based pasta salads, marinated vegetable salads, and plain fruit or fruit cocktail are better salad choices than mayonnaise- or sour cream-based salads such as potato salad, cole slaw, tuna salad, or fruit ambrosia. Some salad bars even classify chocolate whipped cream sprinkled with chocolate chips as a salad.

Delis and Cafeterias

Cafeterias and delis often offer a wider variety of quick but healthful foods than fast food restaurants. You also have more control over portion sizes, added sauces, and dressings. Choose sandwiches made with whole-grain bread, lean meats, and plenty of vegetables such as lettuce, tomato, and onion. Hold the mayonnaise, and ask that the meat be limited to two ounces instead of piled high. Other good deli and cafeteria choices include bean salads, green leafy salads, fresh fruits, vegetarian pizza, and broth-based soups.

JIM'S DIARY: Gay and I have lunch most Sundays at Morrison's Cafeteria. I have a tossed salad with dressing on the side, a bean dish (pinto, navy, or black-eyed peas), cabbage, spinach greens (which we never have at home), another vegetable, and a bowl of diced fruit. This is one of my favorite meals of the week.

Fast Food Restaurants

Forty percent of the dollars we spend eating out are spent in fast food restaurants, and this market share is growing. While typical fast foods such as burgers and fries do provide certain essential vitamins and minerals, they are known for their high fat, sodium, and calorie content.

An occasional burger and fries won't hurt you, and you can round out what you're missing at fast food restaurants (fruits and vegetables) with other meals and snacks throughout the day. Choose a regular hamburger instead of a double with cheese and special sauce. Even though chicken or fish sandwiches sound healthier, they usually contain more fat and calories than burgers because they are breaded and fried.

JIM'S DIARY: Once or twice a month I have an evening church meeting and have to grab a quick snack on the way. McDonald's is convenient, and I often stop there for my fast food. I usually have a chicken fajita or McLean hamburger, McDonaldland cookies, and iced tea. I could make healthier choices but enjoy these and get out with a low-fat meal. By the way, this is much lower in fat and calories than the southern-style meal the church serves.

Fortunately, many fast food restaurants are responding to consumer demand for healthier fare. Major fast food chains now offer whole-grain buns, baked potatoes, salads (watch the toppings and dressings), low-fat milk, and fruit juices. While most fast foods still contain lots of extra fat and calories, we have listed the better choices for some major fast food chains on the next two pages. All of the items listed are for one standard order unless otherwise indicated.

FAST FOOD CHOICES

	Calories	% Calories as Fat		Calories	% Calories as Fat
AVAILABLE WIDELY			**BURGER KING**		
Breakfast:			Chicken salad*	142	25
Bagel, 1	163	8	Chicken sandwich, broiled	267	27
Bran muffin, 1	200	25	Potato, baked, plain,	210	0
Cereal (e.g., Wheaties)	85	10	Salad, side*	25	0
English muffin, 1	135	7	**DAIRY QUEEN/BRAZIER**		
Fruit juice, 6 oz.	80	0	BBQ beef sandwich	225	16
Milk, low-fat, 8 oz.	110	16	Chicken fillet sandwich	300	24
Pancakes, plain, 3	300	10	**DOMINO'S PIZZA**		
Later in the Day:			Cheese pizza, 2 slices	376	24
Chicken sandwich, not fried	280	28	Ham pizza, 2 slices	417	24
Fruit	variable	0	**DUNKIN' DONUTS**		
Potato, baked, plain*	250	0	Bagels, all	240	4
Salad, side*	25	0	Muffins, all	320	26
Vegetables	variable	0	**HARDEE'S**		
ARBY'S			Breakfast:		
Breakfast:			Pancakes, plain, 3	280	6
Blueberry muffin	200	25	Later in the Day:		
Cinnamon nut Danish	340	25	Roast beef sandwich	350	28
Later in the Day:			Chicken 'n' pasta salad*	230	12
Potato, baked, plain	240	0	Chicken sandwich, grilled	310	26
Light roast beef deluxe	296	30	**KFC (Kentucky Fried Chicken)**		
Light roast chicken deluxe	253	17	Beans, baked	133	11
Light roast turkey deluxe	260	21	Corn-on-the-cob	90	20
Salad, side*	25	0	Potatoes, mashed w/gravy	71	25
Soup, beef w/ vegetables					
& barley	96	28			
Soup, chicken noodle	99	18			
Soup, tomato Florentine	84	21			

* No sauce or dressing

FAST FOOD CHOICES

	Calories	% Calories as Fat		Calories	% Calories as Fat
LONG JOHN SILVER'S			**SUBWAY**		
Chicken sandwich, baked	320	23	Salad, garden, large	46	10
Green Beans	30	0	Ham sandwich, 6"	260	28
Seafood, baked cod	150	6	Roast beef sandwich, 6"	375	25
Salad, ocean chef*	150	30	Seafood & crab		
Salad, seafood*	230	20	sandwich, 6"	388	29
Salad, side*	25	0	Subway club sandwich, 6"	379	26
MCDONALD'S			Tuna sandwich, 6"	402	28
Breakfast:			Turkey sandwich, 6"	357	26
Cereal	85	10	Veggies & cheese		
English muffin w/margarine	170	21	sandwich, 6"	268	29
Hotcakes w/margarine			**TACO BELL**		
& syrup	410	20	Burrito, bean & red sauce	447	28
Muffins, all	180	0	**WENDY'S**		
Later in the Day:			Chicken sandwich, grilled	320	25
Carrot sticks	37	0	Chili, 9 oz.	220	29
Chicken sandwich, grilled	252	14	Fettucini, 2 oz.	190	14
McLean deluxe	320	28	Flour tortilla	110	25
Salad, chunky chicken	150	24	Fruit (cantelope, etc.)	variable	0
Salad, side	30	30	Pasta medley, 2 oz.	60	30
PIZZA HUT			Potato, baked, plain	270	0
Salad bar	variable	variable	Rotini, 2 oz.	90	20
			Salad, garden	70	26
			Spanish rice, 2 oz.	70	13
			Turkey ham, ¼ cup	35	25
			Vegetables	variable	0

* No sauce or dressing

Full-Service Restaurants

Full-service restaurants usually offer the greatest variety and flexibility of dining options. You can individually tailor your order and make special requests to meet your needs. Full-service restaurants, however, also serve drinks before meals, wine with the meal, appetizers, desserts, and many other extras in addition to the main course. All this food served in a leisurely, relaxed environment makes it easy to eat and drink much more than you realize.

To avoid filling up on fat-laden foods unintentionally, look for salads, grains, fruits, and vegetables on the menu. When you order these foods, you won't have to worry about how much you eat. Bread is a pretty good choice if you count the number of pieces and leave the butter alone. (To make a point, I often refer to butter or eggs as "the yellow death." I'm a lot of fun at a dinner party!) And remember, you don't have to eat everything just because it's served to you. You might even order an extra plate to split an entree. Focus on the fellowship and atmosphere when you eat out, and enjoy your meal.

JIM'S DIARY: Each Friday night, Gay and I have dinner at a local restaurant. My favorites, listed in order of preference, are: Italian, Mexican, seafood, Continental, Thai, and Chinese. When traveling, I try to find a good sushi bar since Japanese is my absolute favorite. I'll share with you my choices—good, bad, and indifferent—at these restaurants.

The sections that follow give healthful suggestions for different types of restaurants. Since preparation techniques vary from restaurant to restaurant, however, be sure to ask how the food is prepared and make special requests when appropriate. I recommend the GOOD CHOICES for low-fat eating. The HIGHER FAT CHOICES should be avoided; they are listed here to help you identify the gremlins.

American

GOOD CHOICES
- Shrimp cocktail
- Bean soup
- Salad with low-fat dressing
  on the side
- Baked potato with chives
- Fresh vegetables
- Charbroiled chicken
- Baked or broiled fish
- Shish kebab

HIGHER FAT CHOICES
(*not recommended*)
- Most chicken items
- Most beef items
- Most pork items

JIM'S DIARY: I don't seek out American restaurants but, being a good sport, I enjoy ordering intelligently at one. A bean soup is a good starter, a salad with dressing on the side, rolls, baked fish (I tell the server I'm allergic to fat and would appreciate the chef using no fat on my fish), a baked potato with chives and pepper, and a fruit cup.

Chinese

GOOD CHOICES
- Won ton, sizzling rice, subgum,
  or hot and sour soup
- Beef, chicken, or shrimp with
  vegetable dishes
- Teriyaki beef or chicken
- Steamed rice

HIGHER FAT CHOICES
(*not recommended*)
- Fried won tons
- Egg rolls
- Peking duck
- Sweet and sour shrimp, chicken,
  or pork

JIM'S DIARY: I have won ton soup, hot shrimp and vegetables over white rice, and a fortune cookie. When I'm extra hungry, I order a vegetable dish as well. I ask them to use a "dry" wok and no oil at all.

French

GOOD CHOICES
- Vegetable mélange
- Spinach salad
- Grilled shrimp
- Honey-glazed lamb
- Poached salmon
- Huîtres fraîches

HIGHER FAT CHOICES
(*not recommended*):
- Escargots
- French onion soup
- Beef Wellington
- Stuffed shrimp

JIM'S DIARY: I have shrimp cocktail, rolls without butter, salad with dressing on the side, poached fish without sauce, vegetables, and fresh berries topped with brown sugar.

Indian

GOOD CHOICES
- Shrimp or vegetable biryani
- Chapati
- Kulcha
- Naan
- Mulligatawny
- Curried chick peas
- Pullao
- Chicken tikka
- Chicken tandoor
- Fish or chicken masala
- Fish, beef, or chicken vindaloo
- Kheema matter

HIGHER FAT CHOICES
(*not recommended*)
- Coconut soup
- Shami kebab
- Cheese pakoras
- Fried shrimp with poori
- Shrimp malai
- Chicken kandhari
- Beef korma

JIM'S DIARY: I have a curried vegetable appetizer, crackers and bread, a spicy chicken dish, and a fruit dessert.

Italian

GOOD CHOICES
- Steamed clams
- Minestrone or pasta soup
- Bread sticks
- Pasta or shrimp marinara
- Chicken or shrimp primavera
- Chicken or veal cacciatore

HIGHER FAT CHOICES
(*not recommended*)
- Alfredo sauce
- Italian sausage
- Buttered garlic bread

JIM'S DIARY: I have steamed mussels, bread, salad with dressing on the side, rolls without butter, tortellini, and cappuccino.

Japanese

GOOD CHOICES
- Su-udon
- Miso soup
- Suimono
- Seafood sunomono
- Grilled scallops
- Sushi
- Sashimi
- Sukiyaki
- Nebemono
- Yosenabe
- Teriyaki
- Shabu shabu

HIGHER FAT CHOICES
(*not recommended*)
- Tempura
- Agemono

JIM'S DIARY: I have twenty pieces of sushi including tuna, salmon, yellow tail, shrimp, vegetable items, and a handroll. When not having sushi, I have miso soup, salad, grilled fish, and a small dish of ice cream.

Mexican

GOOD CHOICES
- Black bean or tortilla soup
- Black beans
- Bean burritos
- Soft tacos
- Enchiladas
- Tamales
- Gazpacho
- Fajitas
- Chili
- Taco salad
- Mexican rice

HIGHER FAT CHOICES
(*not recommended*)
- Dishes with lots of sour cream or cheese
- Fried tortillas
- Taco chips
- Tostadas
- Quesadillas
- Chimichangas

JIM'S DIARY: I have chips and salsa, tortilla soup, and bean burritos or shrimp fajitas. The chips are my major problem.

Middle Eastern

GOOD CHOICES
- Tabooli
- Hummus
- Couscous
- Dolma
- Pita bread
- Lentil soup
- Rice pilaf
- Gyros
- Shish kebab
- Kibbeh
- Sheikel mashi

HIGHER FAT CHOICES
(*not recommended*)
- Mousaka
- Spanikopita
- Falafel
- Pasticchio
- Baklava

JIM'S DIARY: I have lentil soup, salad, pita bread, and shish kebab. I have an occasional falafel for lunch.

Seafood

GOOD CHOICES
- Oysters or clams on the half shell
- Shrimp or crab cocktail
- Most baked or broiled fish if
    not breaded or stuffed

HIGHER FAT CHOICES
    (*not recommended*)
- Deep fried fish or seafood
- Hush puppies
- Most steaks

JIM'S DIARY: I have oysters on the half shell with plenty of horseradish, salad with salad dressing on the side, rolls without butter, and broiled or blackened fish.

Thai

GOOD CHOICES
- Steamed mussels
- Pad jay
- Crystal noodle
- Seafood kebab
- Pok taek
- Talay sian
- Poy sian
- Scallops bamboo
- Garlic shrimp
- Thai chicken

HIGHER FAT CHOICES
    (*not recommended*)
- Praram long song
- Fried tofu
- Hot Thai catfish
- Crispy duck
- Curried spareribs

JIM'S DIARY: I have a spicy chicken and peanut oil appetizer (high fat, but small serving), the Red Sea, which is spicy shrimp and vegetables with white rice.

Chapter Action Plan

• Tips for Eating Out:

Brown Bag: vegetables, lean meat sandwich, juice, fruit

Traveling: low-fat airline meal, fruit, pretzels, vegetables

Vending: lean meat sandwich, juice, pretzels, animal crackers

Salad Bar: greens, vegetables, beans, fruit

Deli: lean meat on whole-grain bread, fruit

Fast Food: plain baked potato, salad, lean meat, cheese pizza, baked fish

Full-Service Restaurant:

Appetizer—shrimp cocktail, fruit cup, steamed mussels

Soup—bean or lentil, minestrone, won ton, clear soups

Bread—whole-grain, plain rolls without butter

Salad—greens with dressing on the side

Entree—baked fish, vegetable plate or extra vegetables, pasta with red sauce

Dessert—fruit cup, sorbet, or fruit ice

I Can Do That!

- Circle the areas where most of your unwanted fat slips in:

    - Brown bag   - Delis
    - Traveling   - Fast food restaurants
    - Vending machines   - Full-service restaurants
    - Salad bars

- Review the related sections in this chapter.

- Write down what you will do next time.
  (For example: *At fast food restaurants, I will have baked seafood, a side salad with dressing on the side, and a breadstick.*)

_____

_____

_____

_____

_____

_____

_____

_____

_____

_____

_____

I Can Do That! Worksheet

Diet (*circle yes or no*)

    yes   no   eat one serving of cereal daily

    yes   no   eat two servings of fruit daily

    yes   no   eat three servings of vegetables daily

    yes   no   eat four servings of starches daily

Exercise (*choose one*)

    _____ walk twelve miles weekly

    _____ walk twenty miles weekly

    _____ walk thirty to thirty-five miles weekly

Moderation (*circle yes or no*)

    yes   no   avoid cigarettes

    yes   no   drink no more than seven alcoholic drinks weekly

    yes   no   avoid sleeping pills and tranquilizers

    yes   no   avoid "workaholic" behavior

Rest and Relaxation (*circle yes or no*)

    yes   no   get adequate sleep (at least seven hours nightly)

    yes   no   spend two hours quality time with family or friends weekly

    yes   no   take a nap or read for two hours every weekend

    yes   no   take a fun three-day weekend every three months

    yes   no   take a one-week restful vacation yearly

Your signature   Date   Signature of relative or friend

(*Keep this copy for your records.*)

I Can Do That! Worksheet

Diet (*circle yes or no*)

    yes   no   eat one serving of cereal daily

    yes   no   eat two servings of fruit daily

    yes   no   eat three servings of vegetables daily

    yes   no   eat four servings of starches daily

Exercise (*choose one*)

    _____ walk twelve miles weekly

    _____ walk twenty miles weekly

    _____ walk thirty to thirty-five miles weekly

Moderation (*circle yes or no*)

    yes   no   avoid cigarettes

    yes   no   drink no more than seven alcoholic drinks weekly

    yes   no   avoid sleeping pills and tranquilizers

    yes   no   avoid "workaholic" behavior

Rest and Relaxation (*circle yes or no*)

    yes   no   get adequate sleep (at least seven hours nightly)

    yes   no   spend two hours quality time with family or friends weekly

    yes   no   take a nap or read for two hours every weekend

    yes   no   take a fun three-day weekend every three months

    yes   no   take a one-week restful vacation yearly

_____ _____ _____
Your signature   Date   Signature of relative or friend

To receive a free copy of the HCF Prevention Newsletter, tear out this worksheet and mail to HCF Nutrition Foundation, P.O. Box 22124, Lexington, KY 40522, along with your name and address.

RECIPES

APPETIZERS, BEVERAGES, AND SNACKS

Chili Bean Dip

1 15- to 16-ounce can kidney beans, drained
—save juice
4 teaspoons tomato juice
1 tablespoon cider vinegar
1 teaspoon Worcestershire sauce
2 garlic cloves, chopped
2 teaspoons chili powder (to taste)
dash of cayenne pepper
   or liquid red pepper sauce
2 ounces (½ cup) cubed Cheddar cheese
salt (to taste)
black pepper (to taste)
chives (for garnish)

Place first seven ingredients in blender; cover and blend on high until smooth. Add bean juice if mixture is too thick. Add cheese; blend until smooth. Season with salt and pepper as desired. Pour into the top of a double boiler or a very heavy saucepan and heat until hot (or bake at 350 degrees for 15 to 20 minutes or until thoroughly heated). Sprinkle chives on top. Makes 30 1-tablespoon servings.

Variations: For a chunkier dip, mash the beans with a fork, leaving small pieces.

Adjust hotness of dip by varying chili powder and pepper.

Serve with corn chips, vegetables, or pita bread

Per Serving:
calories 20
carbohydrates 3 g
protein 1 g
fat 0 g
saturated fat 0 g
cholesterol 2 mg
sodium 65 mg
fiber 1 g
soluble fiber 0 g

Gingered Fruit Dip

1 cup low-fat cottage cheese
1 small banana, sliced
⅛ teaspoon ground ginger
1 tablespoon skim milk
orange peel cut into thin 2-inch strips

In a blender or food processor combine cottage cheese, banana, and ground ginger. Cover and blend until smooth. Blend in milk. Transfer to an airtight container and chill. Garnish dip with orange peel and serve with fresh fruit dippers. Makes 20 1-tablespoon servings.

Serve with apple wedges, kiwi fruit slices, or mandarin orange sections.

Per Serving:
calories 14
carbohydrate 2 g
protein 1 g
fat 0 g
saturated fat 0 g
cholesterol 1 mg
sodium 46 mg
fiber 0 g
soluble fiber 0 g

Yogurt Vegetable Dip

1 package dry vegetable soup mix
8 ounces plain nonfat yogurt
1 packet Nutrasweet (optional)

In a small bowl, blend vegetable soup mix and Nutrasweet with yogurt. Chill for 2 hours. Serve as dip for vegetables or crackers. Makes 16 1-tablespoon servings.

Variations: Also makes a nice cracker spread.

Serve with broccoli and cauliflower florets, carrot sticks, celery stalks, and/or radishes.

Per Serving:
calories 14
carbohydrate 2 g
protein 1 g
fat 0 g
saturated fat 0 g
cholesterol 0 mg
sodium 110 mg
fiber 0 g
soluble fiber 0 g

Zingy Apple Punch

2 quarts apple juice
1 apple, cut into
  ¼-inch rounds
6 whole cloves
6 allspice berries

1 cinnamon stick
4 Celestial Seasonings
  Red Zinger tea bags
cinnamon sticks (garnish)
thin lemon slices (garnish)

Per Serving:
  calories 120
carbohydrate 30 g
  protein 0 g
  fat 0 g
saturated fat 0 g
cholesterol 0 mg
  sodium 15 mg
  fiber 2 g
soluble fiber 0 g

Pour the apple juice into a 3-quart saucepan. Stick the cloves into the apple slices and add them to the pan. Add the all-spice berries and cinnamon stick. Cover and heat on medium-low until the mixture simmers. Remove from the heat and add the tea bags. Cover the saucepan and steep for 15 minutes. Remove the bags before serving. Ladle into mugs and garnish with a cinnamon stick and lemon slice. Makes 8 1-cup servings.

Tangy Tomato Drink

2 cups tomato juice
⅓ cup water
1 teaspoon sugar
1 teaspoon instant
  beef bouillon
¼ teaspoon celery salt

1 teaspoon lemon juice
dash Worcestershire sauce
dash cayenne pepper
4 celery sticks, about
  5 inches long

Per Serving:
  calories 25
carbohydrate 6 g
  protein 1 g
  fat 0 g
saturated fat 0 g
cholesterol 0 mg
  sodium 650 mg
  fiber 1 g
soluble fiber 0 g

Chill tomato juice. Combine water, sugar, bouillon, and celery salt in 1-cup microwave dish. Microwave, uncovered, on high 1½ to 2 minutes or until boiling; stir to dissolve bouillon. Mix in lemon juice, Worcestershire sauce, and pepper. Blend with chilled juice. Refrigerate until serving. Garnish with celery sticks. Serves 4.

Variations: Celery seed may be substituted for celery salt.

BEANS AND RICE

New Orleans Beans and Rice

½ cup uncooked brown rice
1 teaspoon canola oil
1 cup chopped onions
½ cup diced celery
½ cup diced green pepper
1 15- to 16-ounce can red kidney beans
   (New Orleans Style)
¼ teaspoon hot sauce (to taste)
⅛ teaspoon black pepper
1 teaspoon green chilies (optional)

Per Serving:
calories 135
carbohydrate 26 g
protein 6 g
fat 1 g
saturated fat 0 g
cholesterol 0 mg
sodium 310 mg
fiber 7 g
soluble fiber 3 g

Cook rice as directed. To a large skillet at medium-high heat, add oil and onion and brown for 2 minutes. Turn heat to low and add celery and green peppers; simmer for about 10 minutes. Add beans and seasonings. Bring to a boil, cover, and simmer 5 minutes. Add cooked rice and mix lightly. Add a little water if mixture is too dry. Serves 6.

Tips: Quick-cooking rice will shorten cooking time. The vegetables can be added to the same cooking pan as soon as the rice is done.

Variations: Substitute seasoned pinto beans or black-eyed peas for the kidney beans, then season with 2 teaspoons picante sauce.

Jim's Spicy Baked Beans

2 15- to 16-ounce cans pork and beans
1 green pepper, chopped
½ cup onions, chopped
¼ cup tomato paste or catsup
¼ cup brown sugar
1 tablespoon dry mustard
¼ teaspoon black pepper
⅛ teaspoon ground cloves
⅛ teaspoon cinnamon
4 slices bacon (optional)

Per Serving:
calories 180
carbohydrate 32 g
protein 7 g
fat 3 g
saturated fat 1 g
cholesterol 2 mg
sodium 550 mg
fiber 6 g
soluble fiber 2 g

Mix all ingredients except bacon in 1½-quart casserole. Bake, uncovered, at 350 degrees for 1½ hours. Place bacon in baking dish lined with white paper towels and cover with paper towels. Microwave on high for 3 to 3½ minutes or until crisp. Remove from paper towels quickly. Crumble bacon over baked beans before serving. May be served hot or cold. Serves 8.

Microwave Instructions: Cover casserole dish. Microwave on high for 10 minutes or until slightly bubbly. Stir twice during cooking. Top with bacon as directed above.

Beans and Cranberries

1 16-ounce can whole-berry cranberry sauce
1 15- to 16-ounce can pork and beans, drained
1 15- to 16-ounce can pinto beans, drained
1 15- to 16-ounce can great northern beans, drained
1 cup onions, chopped
4 teaspoons dry mustard

Serve with barbecue main dishes.

continued

Place cranberry sauce in 2-quart microwave casserole dish and break up with a fork. Add beans, onions, and mustard and stir together. Cover dish and microwave on high, stirring every 5 minutes, for 10 to 15 minutes until onions are tender. Let stand for 5 to 10 minutes. Serves 12.

Variations: May be served hot or cold. Three 16-ounce cans of pork and beans or other combinations of canned beans may be used.

Per Serving:
calories 265
carbohydrate 56 g
protein 9 g
fat 1 g
saturated fat 0 g
cholesterol 0 mg
sodium 210 mg
fiber 8 g
soluble fiber 3 g

Savory Black Beans with Tomatoes

1 teaspoon canola oil
1 medium onion, chopped
2 garlic cloves, chopped
1 14- to 16-ounce can tomatoes, drained and chopped
1 15- to 16-ounce can black beans, drained
½ teaspoon tabasco sauce
1 teaspoon cilantro

Very good served over rice.

Heat oil in medium skillet over moderately high heat; add onions and garlic. Sauté, stirring until onion is browned, about 2 to 3 minutes. Add tomatoes and cook, stirring frequently, for 2 minutes more. Add black beans and tabasco sauce; stir. Cover skillet and cook until beans are heated through, about 2 minutes. Remove from heat and stir in cilantro. Serve immediately. Serves 4.

Per Serving:
calories 150
carbohydrate 27 g
protein 8 g
fat 1 g
saturated fat 0 g
cholesterol 0 mg
sodium 300 mg
fiber 9 g
soluble fiber 4 g

Variations: Black-eyed peas, pinto, navy, or kidney beans may be used instead of black beans. Chopped fresh coriander (1 tablespoon) may be used instead of cilantro. Use 2 cups fresh tomatoes when in season. Cajun hot sauce may be substituted for tabasco sauce.

Curried Lentils

2 15½-ounce cans chicken broth
1 cup lentils
1 tablespoon lemon juice
2 teaspoons curry powder (or more, to taste)
1 cup carrots, diced
1 small onion, finely chopped
2 garlic cloves, finely minced
½ teaspoon ground cumin
½ teaspoon chili powder
freshly ground black pepper (to taste)
chopped fresh parsley (garnish)

In a medium saucepan bring broth to a boil. Add the lentils, cover, reduce heat, and simmer slowly for 45 minutes or until lentils are tender. Dissolve curry powder in lemon juice. Add all ingredients except parsley to lentils, stir well, cover, and simmer for an additional 10 to 15 minutes. Serve hot, garnished with parsley. Serves 4.

Variations: Add tomato paste or fresh tomatoes.

May be served as an appetizer.

Per Serving:
calories 145
carbohydrate 21 g
protein 11 g
fat 2 g
saturated fat 0 g
cholesterol 1 mg
sodium 650 mg
fiber 5 g
soluble fiber 2 g

Limed Beans with Green Chilies

1 teaspoon canola oil
½ medium onion, chopped
1 teaspoon lime juice
¼ cup (2 ounces) canned green chilies, minced
½ teaspoon salt (to taste)
1 15- to 16-ounce can pinto beans, rinsed and drained
freshly ground black pepper

Heat oil in medium sauce pan, sauté onion for 2 minutes. Stir in lime juice, minced chilies, and salt. Raise heat to simmer and add the beans and pepper; toss gently. Cook, stirring occasionally, for 2 to 3 minutes or until beans are heated through. Serves 4.

Variations: This also makes a great filling for a burrito.

Serve with baked chicken.

Per Serving:
calories 195
carbohydrate 35 g
protein 10 g
fat 2 g
saturated fat 0 g
cholesterol 0 mg
sodium 250 mg
fiber 7 g
soluble fiber 3 g

Unfried Beans

2 tablespoons finely chopped onion
1 tablespoon ketchup
1 15- to 16-ounce can hot and spicy chili beans

Mix onions and ketchup in small microwave bowl and microwave for 1 minute on high. Put beans in microwave bowl and mash with fork or potato masher. Combine onion mixture with beans; microwave on high 2 minutes. Serves 4.

Variations: One minced garlic clove can be added to enhance taste.

Serve as a side dish or as burrito filling.

Per Serving:
calories 110
carbohydrate 20 g
protein 7 g
fat 0 g
saturated fat 0 g
cholesterol 0 mg
sodium 400 mg
fiber 7 g
soluble fiber 3 g

Cajun Rice

1 cup uncooked regular rice
2 teaspoons canola oil
1 large onion, chopped
1 large green pepper, chopped
4 garlic cloves, minced
1 14½-ounce can stewed tomatoes, undrained
1 cube chicken bouillon
½ teaspoon hot pepper sauce

Cook rice as directed. In medium skillet heat oil over medium-high heat. Stir in onion, pepper, and garlic. Sauté 3 minutes. Stir in rice, tomatoes, bouillon, and hot pepper sauce, breaking tomatoes with a spoon. Bring to boil. Reduce heat; cover and simmer, stirring occasionally for 8 to 10 minutes to blend flavors. Serves 8.

Per Serving:
calories 175
carbohydrate 35 g
protein 4 g
fat 2 g
saturated fat 0 g
cholesterol 0 mg
sodium 370 mg
fiber 3 g
soluble fiber 1 g

Fruit 'n' Rice

3 cups cooked brown rice
1 cup sliced carrots
2 teaspoons canola oil
1 cup sliced green onions
2 cups sliced, cored unpeeled apples
½ cup seedless raisins
1 tablespoon sesame seeds

Cook rice as directed. Sauté carrots in oil about 10 minutes. Add onions and apples. Cook 10 minutes longer; stir in rice and raisins. Cook, stirring constantly, until the rice is heated through. Add sesame seeds and toss lightly. Serves 6.

Per Serving:
calories 155
carbohydrate 32 g
protein 3 g
fat 2 g
saturated fat 0 g
cholesterol 0 mg
sodium 10 mg
fiber 4 g
soluble fiber 1 g

Rice Mexicano

1 cup uncooked long-grain rice
1 tablespoon olive oil
1 small onion, chopped
½ cup green peppers, chopped
½ teaspoon salt
2 teaspoons chili powder (to taste)
1 cup canned tomatoes, undrained

Cook rice as directed. Heat a large skillet to medium-high heat and sauté onions in oil for 2 minutes. Add remaining ingredients, except rice, and cook on medium for 4 minutes. Mix in rice, cover and simmer for 8 to 10 minutes to thoroughly heat rice and blend flavors. Serves 6.

Per Serving:
calories 165
carbohydrate 32 g
protein 3 g
fat 3 g
saturated fat 0 g
cholesterol 0 mg
sodium 300 mg
fiber 2 g
soluble fiber 1 g

Rapid Rice Pilaf

1 teaspoon canola oil
1 green onion, sliced (including top)
¾ cup water
1 teaspoon instant chicken bouillon
¾ cup quick-cooking rice
½ teaspoon parsley flakes
1 tablespoon slivered almonds (optional)

Microwave oil and green onion on high in uncovered 1-quart microwave casserole 45 to 60 seconds or until tender. Add water and bouillon, cover and microwave on high 2½ to 3 minutes or until mixture boils. Add rice and parsley. Cover and let stand 5 minutes. Microwave for 2 minutes until rice is tender. Fluff with fork. Sprinkle with almonds. Serves 3.

Serve with baked chicken, green beans, and rolls.

Per Serving:
calories 105
carbohydrate 20 g
protein 2 g
fat 2 g
saturated fat 0 g
cholesterol 0 mg
sodium 320 mg
fiber 1 g
soluble fiber 0 g

Rice and Mushroom Pilaf

2 teaspoons canola oil
½ cup chopped onion
2 cups sliced mushrooms
1½ cups uncooked converted rice
3½ cups boiling water
¼ teaspoon salt (to taste)
¼ teaspoon black pepper
¼ cup chopped parsley

In heavy medium sauce pan, heat oil until hot and bubbly. Add onion and sauté 5 minutes or until soft. Add mushrooms and cook, stirring frequently, 5 minutes or until tender. Stir in rice until well coated. Add remaining ingredients except parsley. Bring to a boil over high heat. Reduce to low; cover and simmer 20 minutes or until rice is tender. Sprinkle with parsley before serving. Serves 6.

Variations: The rice may be prepared as directed and added to the onion and mushroom mixture after they are cooked. Omit the boiling water and heat for 6 to 10 minutes until thoroughly heated.

Serve with Chicken à l'Orange in Main Dish section.

Per Serving:
calories 195
carbohydrate 40 g
protein 4 g
fat 2 g
saturated fat 0 g
cholesterol 0 mg
sodium 80 mg
fiber 2 g
soluble fiber 1 g

Savory Brown Rice

1 cup uncooked brown rice
1 tablespoon canola oil
2 green onions with tops, thinly sliced
1 teaspoon caraway seeds
1 cinnamon stick
1 cup chicken broth
1½ cups water

In 2- or 3-quart saucepan, heat oil over medium-high heat. Add onions, caraway, and cinnamon. Sauté, stirring frequently, until onions are soft, about 3 minutes. Stir in the rice and sauté for an additional minute. Add broth and water; bring mixture to a boil. Reduce heat and simmer, covered, 30 to 40 minutes or until rice is tender and liquid is absorbed. Fluff rice with fork, remove cinnamon stick, and serve immediately. Serves 4.

Variations: The rice may be prepared separately according to instructions and added as indicated. Do not add water; simmer for 8 to 10 minutes to blend flavors.

Per Serving:
calories 125
carbohydrate 19 g
protein 3 g
fat 4 g
saturated fat 0 g
cholesterol 0 mg
sodium 190 mg
fiber 2 g
soluble fiber 0 g

BREADS AND MUFFINS

Parmesan Italian Bread

1 small loaf French bread (about 8 ounces)
2 ounces Neufchâtel cheese
2 tablespoons grated Parmesan cheese
1 tablespoon snipped chives
1 tablespoon snipped parsley
⅛ teaspoon garlic powder

Cut bread in half lengthwise, cutting to, but not through, crust; set aside. Microwave Neufchâtel cheese on high in uncovered 1-cup microwave measure 30 to 45 seconds or until softened. Stir in remaining ingredients. Spread mixture on cut side of bottom piece of bread. Replace with top. Wrap in paper toweling. Place in plastic bag and refrigerate.

To serve, remove bread from plastic bag and microwave on high 45 to 60 seconds or until bread feels warm. Serves 8.

Goes well with spaghetti or salad.

Per Serving:
calories 105
carbohydrate 15 g
protein 4 g
fat 3 g
saturated fat 2 g
cholesterol 7 mg
sodium 210 mg
fiber 1 g
soluble fiber 0 g

Dijon French Bread

½ of a 16-ounce loaf of French bread
1 tablespoon canola oil
1 tablespoon Dijon mustard
1 tablespoon minced fresh parsley
⅛ teaspoon black pepper

Slice bread in half lengthwise, leaving one side attached. Open bread, butterfly fashion; set aside. Combine oil, mustard, parsley, and pepper in a small bowl; stir well. Spread mixture over cut sides of bread. Reassemble loaf and wrap tightly in aluminum foil. Bake at 350 degrees for 15 minutes or until thoroughly heated. Cut bread into 8 1-inch slices. Serves 8.

Per Slice:
calories 100
carbohydrate 15 g
protein 3 g
fat 3 g
saturated fat 0 g
cholesterol 0 mg
sodium 180 mg
fiber 1 g
soluble fiber 0 g

Hearty Oat-Corn Bread

1 cup uncooked rolled oats (quick or old fashioned)
1 cup corn meal
½ cup all-purpose flour
2 tablespoons sugar
1 tablespoon baking powder
¼ teaspoon salt (optional)
1 cup skim milk
½ cup frozen kernel corn, thawed
2 tablespoons canola oil
2 egg whites, slightly beaten
2 tablespoons finely chopped onion

Heat oven to 425 degrees. Lightly oil 8- or 9-inch square baking pan. Combine dry ingredients. Add combined remaining ingredients; mix well. Spread evenly into prepared pan. Bake 20 to 25 minutes or until edges are lightly browned. Serve warm. Cut into 9 slices.

Tasty when served with bean dishes or barbecue.

Per Slice:
calories 195
carbohydrate 32 g
protein 6 g
fat 5 g
saturated fat 0 g
cholesterol 0 mg
sodium 190 mg
fiber 3 g
soluble fiber 1 g

Microwave Instructions: Prepare batter as directed above. Spread evenly into 8-inch square microwave dish. Microwave at medium-low or medium 6 minutes or until center is set, turning dish once. Let stand 5 minutes before serving.

Tips: If you microwave, you may brown top of cornbread under broiler for a few seconds.

Variations: Add green pepper for Mexican cornbread.

Cinnamon Quick Loaf

2 cups all-purpose flour
1 cup oat bran hot cereal
½ cup firmly packed light brown sugar
1 tablespoon baking powder
1 teaspoon baking soda
1 teaspoon ground cinnamon
1 cup skim milk
½ cup (4 ounces) egg substitute
2 tablespoons canola oil
1 teaspoon vanilla extract

Per Slice:
calories 110
carbohydrate 20 g
protein 3 g
fat 2 g
saturated fat 1 g
cholesterol 0 mg
sodium 140 mg
fiber 1 g
soluble fiber 0 g

In large bowl, combine flour, oat bran, brown sugar, baking powder, baking soda, and cinnamon; set aside. In small bowl, combine milk, egg substitute, oil, and vanilla; stir into dry ingredients just until blended. Spread into greased and floured 9 x 5 x 3-inch loaf pan. Bake at 350 degrees for 45 to 50 minutes or until toothpick inserted in center comes out clean. Remove from pan; cool on wire rack. Cut into 16 slices.

Variations: Make cinnamon, brown sugar, and margarine topping, crumble on top before baking.

Blueberry Banana Bread

¾ cup whole-wheat flour
1 cup all-purpose flour
1 teaspoon baking soda
¼ teaspoon salt
½ teaspoon cinnamon
½ cup quick-cooking rolled oats
2 tablespoons canola oil
⅓ cup sugar
¼ cup (2 ounces) egg substitute
1 cup mashed bananas (about 2 whole)
1 tablespoon lemon juice
1 cup fresh or frozen blueberries, thawed
    (about 4 ounces)

Per Slice:
calories 145
carbohydrate 26 g
protein 3 g
fat 3 g
saturated fat 0 g
cholesterol 0 mg
sodium 140 mg
fiber 2 g
soluble fiber 0 g

Preheat oven to 350 degrees and lightly grease 9 x 5-inch loaf pan. Mix flour, soda, salt, and cinnamon. Stir in oats and set aside. Mix oil and sugar. Whip in egg substitute; add bananas and lemon juice and stir until blended. Fold in blueberries. Add dry ingredients and mix until just moistened. Pour batter in loaf pan and bake for about 1 hour. Let bread cool in pan for 10 minutes. Remove bread from pan and place on wire rack to cool. Wrap and refrigerate several hours before slicing. Cut into 12 slices.

Variations: Use frozen blueberries thawed in microwave. Add all juice to batter also.

Comments: A 2-slice serving contains less than 1½ teaspoons sugar.

Raw Apple Bran Muffins

1¼ cups whole-wheat flour
1 cup oat bran
⅓ cup packed brown sugar
2½ teaspoons baking powder
¼ teaspoon baking soda
¼ teaspoon salt
¼ teaspoon ground nutmeg
¼ teaspoon ground cinnamon
1 cup buttermilk
2 egg whites
2 tablespoons canola oil
¾ cup shredded, peeled apple

Per Muffin:
calories 115
carbohydrate 19 g
protein 3 g
fat 3 g
saturated fat 0 g
cholesterol 1 mg
sodium 160 mg
fiber 2 g
soluble fiber 1 g

In a medium bowl stir together flour, oat bran, brown sugar, baking powder, baking soda, salt, nutmeg, and cinnamon. Set aside. In a small bowl combine buttermilk, egg whites, and oil. Add to dry ingredients; stir just until moistened. Stir in shredded apple. Store batter, tightly covered, in the refrigerator for up to 5 days.

To bake, spray muffin cups with nonstick spray coating. Spoon about ¼ cup batter into each muffin cup. Bake at 375 degrees for 18 to 20 minutes. Makes 12 muffins.

Variations: 1 cup skim milk and 1 teaspoon lemon juice may be substituted for buttermilk.

Applesauce Oat Muffins

1 cup crushed whole-grain oat cereal (e.g., Cheerios;
  approximately 2 cups uncrushed cereal)
1¼ cup all-purpose flour
⅓ cup packed brown sugar
1 teaspoon ground cinnamon
1 teaspoon baking powder
¾ teaspoon baking soda
1 cup applesauce
⅓ cup skim milk
½ cup raisins (optional)
2 tablespoons canola oil
1 egg white
1 tablespoon wheat germ (optional)

Per Muffin:
calories 100
carbohydrate 19 g
protein 2 g
fat 2 g
saturated fat 0 g
cholesterol 0 mg
sodium 110 mg
fiber 1 g
soluble fiber 0 g

Preheat oven to 400 degrees. Spray 12 muffin cups with non-stick spray. In a large bowl, mix cereal, flour, brown sugar, cinnamon, baking powder, and baking soda. Stir in remaining ingredients just until moistened. Divide batter evenly among muffin cups. Bake 18 to 22 minutes or until golden brown. Remove from cups and serve. Makes 12 muffins.

Blueberry Oat Muffins

2½ cups uncooked oats
½ cup firmly packed brown sugar
2 teaspoons baking powder
¼ teaspoon salt (optional)
½ teaspoon cinnamon
1 cup fresh or frozen blueberries
⅔ cup skim milk
2 tablespoons canola oil
2 egg whites, slightly beaten

Per Muffin:
calories 140
carbohydrate 24 g
protein 2 g
fat 4 g
saturated fat 0 g
cholesterol 0 mg
sodium 80 mg
fiber 2 g
soluble fiber 1 g

Heat oven to 400 degrees. Place oats in blender or food processor; cover and blend or process about 1 minute, stopping occasionally to stir. Combine ground oats, brown sugar, baking powder, salt, and cinnamon. Add blueberries, milk, oil, and egg whites, mixing just until moistened. Line 12 medium muffin cups with paper baking cups. Fill muffin cups almost full. Bake 20 to 22 minutes or until deep golden brown. Makes 12 muffins.

May be frozen and reheated in the microwave.

Blueberry Bran Muffins

2⅔ cups All-Bran cereal
1½ cups skim milk
4 egg whites
1 tablespoon vanilla
2 cups flour
⅔ cup brown sugar
2 tablespoons baking powder
¾ teaspoon baking soda
1½ teaspoons cinnamon
2 cups blueberries, fresh or frozen

Preheat oven to 325 degrees. Combine bran cereal, milk, egg whites, and vanilla; let stand 5 minutes. Stir together flour, brown sugar, baking powder, baking soda, and cinnamon in large bowl. Add cereal-milk mixture and mix. Add blueberries and stir carefully. Spoon into lightly oiled or paper-lined muffin tins. Bake 30 minutes. Makes 16 muffins.

May be frozen and reheated in the oven.

Per Muffin:
calories 160
carbohydrate 35 g
protein 5 g
fat 0 g
saturated fat 0 g
cholesterol 0 mg
sodium 350 mg
fiber 5 g
soluble fiber 1 g

Quick & Easy Oatmeal Muffins

¼ cup (2 ounces) egg substitute
¼ cup packed brown sugar
2 tablespoons canola oil
⅓ cup low-fat buttermilk
½ cup unsifted all-purpose flour
¼ cup quick-cooking rolled oats
1 teaspoon baking powder
¼ teaspoon soda
¼ teaspoon salt

Per Muffin:
calories 100
carbohydrate 15 g
protein 3 g
fat 3 g
saturated fat 0 g
cholesterol 0 mg
sodium 170 mg
fiber 0 g
soluble fiber 0 g

Beat egg substitute; blend in sugar, oil, and buttermilk until smooth. Add remaining ingredients; stir just until moistened. Spoon into paper-lined microwave muffin cups, filling half full. Cover and refrigerate up to 24 hours.

To serve, microwave on high 6 muffins at a time, uncovered, 2 to 2½ minutes or until no longer doughy, rotating pan once. For remaining 2 muffins, decrease time to 45 to 50 seconds. Makes 8 muffins.

Tips: When storing batter for longer than 24 hours, refrigerate it in a covered dish and then spoon into muffin cups as needed. When muffins are cooked immediately, decrease time to 1¾ to 2¼ minutes.

Variations: Batter may be sprinkled with toasted wheat germ or cinnamon and sugar before cooking; ⅓ cup skim milk and 1 teaspoon lemon juice may be substituted for buttermilk.

Orange Muffins

1½ cups whole-wheat flour
½ cup oat bran hot cereal
1½ teaspoons baking soda
¾ cup orange juice
¼ cup (2 ounces) egg substitute, beaten
1 teaspoon grated orange rind
¼ cup honey
2 tablespoons canola oil
½ cup raisins

Per Muffin:
calories 130
carbohydrate 24 g
protein 3 g
fat 3 g
saturated fat 0 g
cholesterol 0 mg
sodium 110 mg
fiber 2 g
soluble fiber 1 g

In a large mixing bowl, combine the flour, oat bran cereal, and baking soda. In a separate bowl mix orange juice, egg substitute, orange rind, honey, oil, and raisins; combine with dry ingredients. Fill well-greased or paper-lined muffin cups about ¾ full with batter and bake at 375 degrees for 15 minutes. Makes 12 muffins.

Variations: You may use ¾ cup white flour and ¾ cup whole wheat flour; wheat bran or wheat bran cereal may be substituted for oat bran.

Gay's Pineapple Oat Bran Muffins

2 cups oat bran cereal
½ cup white all-purpose flour
¼ cup brown sugar
1 tablespoon baking powder
½ cup skim milk
1 8-ounce can crushed pineapple in juice
   (unsweetened)
½ cup (4 ounces) egg substitute
2 tablespoons canola oil

Preheat oven to 425 degrees. Mix dry ingredients in a large bowl. Combine milk, pineapple with juice, egg substitute, and oil in a bowl or blender. Add dry ingredients and mix lightly. Spray muffin pans with nonstick spray. Fill muffin cups three-quarters full. Bake 17 minutes. Makes 12 muffins.

Variations: You may add cinnamon to modify the flavor.

May be served hot or cold.

Per Muffin:
calories 112
carbohydrate 18 g
protein 3 g
fat 3 g
saturated fat 0 g
cholesterol 0 mg
sodium 110 mg
fiber 2.2 g
soluble fiber 1.1 g

BREAKFAST FOODS

Allison's French Toast

½ cup (4 ounces) egg substitute
¼ cup water
½ cup skim milk
½ teaspoon vanilla
1 tablespoon brown sugar
cinnamon
6 slices whole-wheat bread

Mix first 5 ingredients together. Spray skillet or griddle with canola nonstick cooking spray and heat. Dip bread in egg mixture one piece at a time, coating both sides. Place on skillet, brown on both sides, and sprinkle each piece with cinnamon. Serves 6.

Variations: For extra cinnamon flavor, sprinkle liberally with cinnamon before putting in skillet. You may also dust with powdered sugar before serving.

Comments: The Allison of the title is my four-year-old granddaughter; we love to make these for the family on Saturday mornings.

Use generous amounts of nonstick spray to keep toast from sticking.

Per Serving:
calories 110
carbohydrate 18 g
protein 6 g
fat 2 g
saturated fat 0 g
cholesterol 0 mg
sodium 230 mg
fiber 2 g
soluble fiber 0 g

Banana Pancakes

1 very ripe medium banana, peeled and
    cut into pieces
¼ cup (2 ounces) egg substitute
1 teaspoon canola oil
½ teaspoon vanilla extract
3 tablespoons all-purpose flour
1 teaspoon double-acting baking powder

Per Serving:
calories 145
carbohydrate 22 g
protein 6 g
fat 4 g
saturated fat 0 g
cholesterol 0 mg
sodium 270 mg
fiber 1 g
soluble fiber 0 g

In blender container combine banana, egg substitute, oil,
and vanilla and blend until smooth; add flour and baking
powder and blend to combine.

Spray 9-inch nonstick skillet with nonstick cooking spray
and heat. Drop 4 heaping tablespoonfuls batter into hot skillet, making 4 pancakes. (Use back of spoon to spread batter
into circles about 3 inches in diameter.) Cook over medium-
high heat until pancakes are browned on bottom and bubbles
appear on surface; turn pancakes and brown other side.
Respray skillet and cook 4 more pancakes. Makes 8 small
pancakes to serve 2.

Comments: Serve with reduced-calorie pancake syrup,
Homemade Maple Syrup (recipe follows), or fruit-flavored
spread such as Apricot Spread (see *Fruits and Desserts*).

Homemade Maple Syrup

½ cup apple juice
2 teaspoons cornstarch
⅓ cup packed brown sugar
¼ cup water
¼ teaspoon maple flavoring

*To reheat syrup,
microwave 45 to
60 seconds.*

Combine juice, cornstarch, brown sugar, and water in 2-cup microwave measure and microwave, uncovered, on high 2 to 3 minutes or until mixture boils and thickens slightly, stirring once. Stir in flavoring. Store in refrigerator. Makes about 12 1-tablespoon servings.

Per Serving:
calories 30
carbohydrate 7 g
protein 0 g
fat 0 g
saturated fat 0 g
cholesterol 0 mg
sodium 2 mg
fiber 0 g
soluble fiber 0 g

Cinnamon Bran Pancakes

¾ cup oat bran
½ cup all-purpose flour
¼ cup whole-wheat flour
1 tablespoon sugar
1 tablespoon baking powder
½ teaspoon ground cinnamon
¼ teaspoon baking soda

⅛ teaspoon salt
2 egg whites, slightly beaten
1¼ cups buttermilk
1 tablespoon canola oil
1 teaspoon vanilla

In medium bowl combine oat bran, flours, sugar, baking powder, cinnamon, soda, and salt. In a small mixing bowl combine egg whites, buttermilk, oil, and vanilla; beat with fork just until combined. Add to dry ingredients, stirring just until combined.

To save time spray the skillet or griddle and heat it while you mix the batter.

Spray a cold griddle or large skillet with nonstick spray coating and heat. For each pancake, spoon ¼ cup of batter onto hot griddle. Cook over medium heat until golden, turning once. Makes 8 to 10 pancakes to serve 4.

Variations: Use equal amounts of white and whole-wheat flour; 1¼ cups skim milk and 1 tablespoon lemon juice may be substituted for buttermilk.

Comments: Whole-grain pancakes take longer to cook but are well worth the wait.

Per Serving:
calories 175
carbohydrate 24 g
protein 8 g
fat 5 g
saturated fat 1 g
cholesterol 3 mg
sodium 470 mg
fiber 3 g
soluble fiber 1 g

Orange 'n' Nut Waffles

½ cup all-purpose flour
½ teaspoon baking powder
¼ teaspoon baking soda
¼ teaspoon ground cinnamon
¼ teaspoon ground nutmeg
⅓ cup buttermilk
¼ cup orange juice
¼ cup (2 ounces) egg substitute
1 teaspoon grated orange peel
1 tablespoon (½ ounce) chopped pecans
2 tablespoons low-calorie pancake syrup
    (14 calories per tablespoon)

Per Serving:
calories 200
carbohydrate 32 g
protein 9 g
fat 4 g
saturated fat 1 g
cholesterol 2 mg
sodium 260 mg
fiber 0 g
soluble fiber 0 g

In medium mixing bowl combine flour, baking powder, baking soda, cinnamon, and nutmeg; set aside.

In small bowl combine buttermilk, orange juice, egg substitute, and orange peel; add to flour mixture and mix well. Mix in pecans. Spray nonstick waffle iron with nonstick cooking spray and preheat.

To serve, cook 4 waffles according to manufacturer's directions for waffle iron and top each with 1 tablespoon syrup. Serves 2.

Tips: Cook waffles in advance, wrap individually, and freeze. Then just pop them in the microwave or toaster-oven to enjoy.

Variations: Chopped walnuts may be substituted for pecans; ⅓ cup skim milk and 1 teaspoon lemon juice may be substituted for buttermilk.

Quick Waffles with Peach Sauce

1 8-ounce can sliced peaches
water
2 teaspoons cornstarch
1 teaspoon lemon juice
⅛ teaspoon ground cinnamon
4 frozen waffles

Drain juice from peaches into 2-cup microwave measure. Add water to make ⅔ cup. Blend in cornstarch, lemon juice, and cinnamon.

Microwave, uncovered, on high 1¼ to 1½ minutes or until mixture boils and thickens, stirring once. Add peaches and set aside. Arrange frozen waffles on microwave serving plate. Microwave, uncovered, on high 1 to 1¼ minutes or until thawed. Top with peach sauce and microwave, uncovered, on high 1½ to 2 minutes or until waffles are heated. Serves 4.

Variations: Microwave the sauce with peaches added for 1¼ minutes and spoon over waffles.

A quick and tasty breakfast.

Per Serving:
calories 125
carbohydrate 21 g
protein 2 g
fat 4 g
saturated fat 1 g
cholesterol 30 mg
sodium 260 mg
fiber 1 g
soluble fiber 0 g

Jim's Breakfast Burrito

2 7½-ounce cartons cholesterol-free vegetable
   omelet mix
½ cup fresh or canned tomatoes, chopped
1 large onion, chopped
¼ green pepper, chopped
2 to 4 tablespoons salsa (to taste)
salt (to taste)
freshly ground black pepper (to taste)
4 10-inch tortillas
½ cup (2 ounces) Cheddar cheese, grated
taco sauce or salsa (optional)

Per Serving:
calories 215
carbohydrate 26 g
protein 17 g
fat 5 g
saturated fat 2 g
cholesterol 8 mg
sodium 260 mg
fiber 2 g
soluble fiber 1 g

Spray medium skillet with canola nonstick cooking spray.
Pour omelet mix, onion, green pepper, and salsa into skillet.
Cook over medium heat until firm, adding salt, pepper, and
additional salsa to taste. Stack the four tortillas between
very moist paper towels and microwave them on high for 2
minutes. Spread tortilla on plate and spoon one-quarter of
the omelet mixture onto left edge of tortilla; sprinkle with
one-quarter of the cheese, roll, and place in glass casserole
pan. Repeat for remaining tortillas. Cover casserole with
moistened paper towels and microwave on high for 2 minutes. Serve with additional salsa or taco sauce. Serves 4.

Tips: Place tortillas between paper towels first and put in
microwave when omelet mix is almost done.

Variations: 1½ cups (12 ounces) of egg substitute may be
used instead of omelet mixture; include ½ green pepper and
½ red pepper, both chopped. Also may be served as Mexican
scrambled eggs.

FRUITS AND DESSERTS

Apricot Spread

3 ounces dried apricots, roughly chopped
⅔ cup unsweetened apple juice

In a small saucepan bring the apricots and juice to a boil. Cover, reduce heat, and simmer very slowly 45 minutes or until smooth and softened, stirring occasionally. Cool mixture slightly, then process in a food processor or blender until smooth. Place in a covered container and chill at least 4 to 6 hours. Serve chilled. Makes 8 1-tablespoon servings.

Variations: Other dried fruits such as peaches or prunes may be substituted for the apricots.

May be used for toast, waffles, and pancakes.

Per Serving:
calories 35
carbohydrate 9 g
protein 0 g
fat 0 g
saturated fat 0 g
cholesterol 0 mg
sodium 2 mg
fiber 0 g
soluble fiber 0 g

Jim's Ambrosia

1 6-ounce can frozen orange juice, undiluted
1 8½-ounce can crushed pineapple, with juice
3 apples, grated
1 banana, mashed
1 cup (4 ounces) grated coconut
¼ cup chopped pecans or walnuts (optional)
8 maraschino cherries

Improves when stored in the refrigerator.

continued

Spoon orange juice into 2-quart bowl. Add pineapple, apples, banana, coconut, and nuts; mix well. Chill for several hours or overnight. Spoon into 8 dessert dishes; top each with a maraschino cherry. Serves 8.

Per Serving:
calories 170
carbohydrate 32 g
protein 2 g
fat 4 g
saturated fat 3 g
cholesterol 0 mg
sodium 30 mg
fiber 4 g
soluble fiber 2 g

Blueberries in Snow

**1 pint fresh blueberries,
washed and cleaned
1 cup plain low-fat yogurt
2 to 3 tablespoons sugar
1 teaspoon vanilla extract
¼ teaspoon almond extract**

Per Serving:
calories 100
carbohydrate 20 g
protein 3 g
fat 1 g
saturated fat 0 g
cholesterol 14 mg
sodium 44 mg
fiber 2 g
soluble fiber 0 g

Place the blueberries in 4 dessert dishes and chill until ready to serve. In a small bowl, whisk yogurt with sugar and extracts. Chill until ready to serve.

To serve, place a dollop of the yogurt mixture on each blueberry dish. Serves 4.

Tips: Blueberries are perishable so they should be used within a few days of purchasing. Refrigerate the berries without rinsing until ready to use. Fresh blueberries work best for this dessert. Frozen blueberries become watery and lose their texture.

Variations: Other fresh berries or peeled and sliced peaches or nectarines may be substituted for the blueberries. Artificial sweetener, 4 to 6 packets, may be substituted for sugar.

Tangy Baked Fruit

1 15¼-ounce can peach halves, with juice
1 15¼-ounce can pear halves, with juice
1 15¼-ounce can pineapple chunks, with juice
1 10-ounce bottle maraschino cherries, with juice
½ cup packed light brown sugar
2 teaspoons curry powder (adjust to taste)

Drain juice from all fruit into 1-quart mixing bowl; add brown sugar and curry powder and mix. Combine fruit in 1½-quart casserole. Spoon juice mixture over fruit, toss lightly, and bake for 1 hour at 350 degrees. Serve warm or refrigerate first. Serves 6.

Tips: May be microwaved for 20 minutes at moderate (60 percent) power.

Variations: Use brown sugar substitute and fruit packed in water to reduce calories. Other fruits such as apricot halves may be substituted.

Improves with age when refrigerated.

Per Serving:
calories 130
carbohydrate 32 g
protein 1 g
fat 0 g
saturated fat 0 g
cholesterol 0 mg
sodium 8 mg
fiber 3 g
soluble fiber 1 g

Wake-Up Fruit Cup

½ medium-sized cantaloupe
2 kiwi fruit
1 pint strawberries
½ pint fresh raspberries or blackberries
2 to 3 tablespoons chopped fresh mint leaves
    plus 4 whole sprigs for garnish
¼ cup orange juice

Freshly squeezed orange juice makes this fruit cup extra special.

continued

Remove seeds from cantaloupe. Scoop out pulp with a melon scoop and place balls in a bowl. Pour any cantaloupe juice in bowl. Peel kiwi. Cut crosswise into thin slices, then quarter the slices and add to cantaloupe.

Set aside 4 attractive strawberries for garnish. Hull and slice remaining strawberries lengthwise; add to bowl. Add raspberries. Sprinkle fruit salad with chopped mint leaves and drizzle with orange juice. Toss gently. Refrigerate, covered, for ½ hour for flavors to blend together.

To serve, divide into 4 bowls. Garnish each with a whole strawberry and a sprig of mint. Serves 4.

Per Serving:
calories 110
carbohydrate 24 g
protein 2 g
fat 1 g
saturated fat 0 g
cholesterol 0 mg
sodium 10 mg
fiber 5 g
soluble fiber 1 g

Blueberry Soup

1½ cups blueberries
1 cup plain low-fat yogurt
½ cup orange juice
2 tablespoons light sour cream
1 tablespoon grated lemon peel
½ teaspoon cinnamon
2 teaspoons artificial sweetener (to taste)

In food processor, combine all ingredients; process until smooth. Chill soup at least 30 minutes before serving. Makes 4 servings.

Per Serving:
calories 95
carbohydrate 16 g
protein 4 g
fat 2 g
saturated fat 1 g
cholesterol 4 mg
sodium 50 mg
fiber 2 g
soluble fiber 0 g

Morning Fruit Kabobs

3¾ cups mixed fruit chunks
1 lime, thinly sliced
½ cup nonfat yogurt
2 teaspoons lime juice
1 teaspoon honey
¼ teaspoon grated nutmeg (to taste)
mint sprigs (garnish)

In large bowl, toss the fruit with the lime slices, then thread on 6-inch skewers. In small bowl, combine yogurt, lime juice, honey, and nutmeg. Drizzle sauce over fruit or serve on the side. Garnish with mint. Serves 4.

Variations: Serve the fruit in a bowl and drizzle the sauce over it.

For extra easy preparation, buy fruit chunks at the supermarket salad bar.

Per Serving:
calories 110
carbohydrate 25 g
protein 2 g
fat 0 g
saturated fat 0 g
cholesterol 1 mg
sodium 20 mg
fiber 2 g
soluble fiber 1 g

Carol's Fruit and Yogurt

2 15¼-ounce cans of tropical fruit salad
½ cup nonfat plain yogurt
1 tablespoon sugar-free instant vanilla pudding

Drain juice from fruit into 1-quart bowl; set fruit aside. Whisk pudding with small amount of yogurt to disperse. Add yogurt and pudding to juice and mix until smooth. Add fruit and mix. Cover and refrigerate 30 minutes or until chilled. Serves 4.

Tips: Have canned fruit and yogurt refrigerated so this tasty dessert will be ready to eat immediately.

Variations: Use any fresh or canned fruit.

Per Serving:
calories 150
carbohydrate 36 g
protein 1 g
fat 0 g
saturated fat 0 g
cholesterol 0 mg
sodium 40 mg
fiber 5 g
soluble fiber 2 g

Overnight Fruit Cup

¼ cup unsweetened orange juice
3 tablespoons sugar
2 teaspoons brown sugar
1½ tablespoons lemon juice
2 tablespoons water
½ teaspoon vanilla extract
1½ cups fresh strawberries,
    cored and quartered
1 cup peeled, sliced peaches
1 cup fresh blueberries

Per Serving:
calories 75
carbohydrate 18 g
protein 1 g
fat 0 g
saturated fat 0 g
cholesterol 0 mg
sodium 5 mg
fiber 2 g
soluble fiber 1 g

Combine first five ingredients in medium saucepan; stir well. Bring to boil; reduce heat and simmer 3 minutes. Remove from heat and stir in vanilla. Combine strawberries, peaches, and blueberries in non-aluminum bowl; pour orange juice mixture over fruit and stir. Cover and refrigerate for at least 8 hours. Serves 6.

Variations: Substitute honeydew melon balls for blueberries. To reduce calories, replace the sugar with artificial sweetener. The orange juice mixture may be mixed in a microwave bowl and microwaved for 1 minute on high.

Gay's Fruit Salad

2 pears, cored and chopped
1 small bunch seedless grapes
   (about 20 large grapes)
2 oranges, peeled and chopped
2 apples, cored and chopped
1 16-ounce can pineapple chunks, drained
2 bananas, chopped or sliced
lemon juice
¼ cup soft tofu
¼ cup plain low-fat yogurt
6 ounce low-fat cherry yogurt
¼ cup chopped pecans or walnuts (optional)

Per Serving:
calories 115
carbohydrate 24 g
protein 2 g
fat 1 g
saturated fat 0 g
cholesterol 2 mg
sodium 20 mg
fiber 3 g
soluble fiber 1 g

Sprinkle apples and bananas with lemon juice. In a very large serving bowl, mix all the fruits together. Process tofu and plain yogurt in a blender until smooth. Stir together with cherry yogurt; pour over fruit. Toss gently. Serve cold. Serves 6.

Variations: ¾ cup raisins or a 7-ounce package grated coconut may be added. Each serving may be topped with a maraschino cherry.

Fruit with Gingered Yogurt Sauce

*May be prepared
the day before.*

2 cups nonfat yogurt
1 tablespoon sugar or to taste
1 teaspoon minced crystallized ginger
12 pineapple rings

In a bowl, combine the yogurt, sugar, and ginger. Place two pineapple rings on each of 6 plates and coat with sauce or serve sauce separately. Serves 6.

Variations: Raspberries may be substituted for pineapple. This sauce is great with a variety of fruits.

Per Serving:
calories 90
carbohydrate 17 g
protein 5 g
fat 0 g
saturated fat 0 g
cholesterol 1 mg
sodium 40 mg
fiber 1 g
soluble fiber 0 g

Gingered Fruit in a Hurry

1 15¼-ounce can tropical fruit salad
¼ teaspoon ginger (to taste)

Empty fruit into mixing bowl. Add ginger and stir until well dispersed. Serves 2.

Tips: If fruit is not chilled, add 6 ice cubes when mixing.

Variations: Use any canned fruit for this quick appetizer, salad, breakfast side dish, or dessert. For fresh fruit, add ¼ cup water and 1 packet of Equal for sweetening.

Comments: Tropical fruit salad is one of my favorites. When I am home alone I usually have this for dessert. Often I put the can in the freezer when I start the meal and have a "slush" for dessert.

Per Serving:
calories 140
carbohydrate 34 g
protein 0 g
fat 0 g
saturated fat 0 g
cholesterol 0 mg
sodium 20 mg
fiber 2 g
soluble fiber 1 g

Sugar-Glazed Grapefruit

2 grapefruit, halved
2 tablespoons brown sugar
2 maraschino cherries, halved (optional)

Remove seeds from grapefruit halves. Cut around sections to loosen. Place on one large or four small microwave plates. Top each half with ½ tablespoon brown sugar; garnish with cherry half. Microwave on high, uncovered, 2 to 3 minutes or until grapefruit are heated and sugar is melted. Serves 4.

Per Serving:
calories 70
carbohydrate 16 g
protein 1 g
fat 0 g
saturated fat 0 g
cholesterol 0 mg
sodium 5 mg
fiber 2 g
soluble fiber 1 g

Frozen Peach Dessert

1 16-ounce can unsweetened sliced peaches,
** well-drained**
1 cup plain nonfat yogurt
1½ tablespoons honey

Place peach slices on a baking sheet, making sure that slices are not touching. Freeze for 1½ hours or until hard.

Remove from freezer and place in chilled food processor or blender. Add yogurt and honey and process until smooth. Spoon into chilled dessert cups and sprinkle with your favorite topping. Serve immediately. Serves 4.

Per Serving:
calories 85
carbohydrate 18 g
protein 4 g
fat 0 g
saturated fat 0 g
cholesterol 1 mg
sodium 50 mg
fiber 2 g
soluble fiber 1 g

Peaches with Cinnamon Top

1 16-ounce can sliced cling peaches, drained
1 teaspoon lemon juice
dash of salt
½ cup frozen lite whipped topping, thawed
¼ teaspoon cinnamon
4 graham cracker squares

About 20 minutes before serving, blend peaches, lemon juice, and salt in a blender at medium speed until smooth; set aside. In a small bowl, stir whipped topping and cinnamon until blended. Crumble graham crackers into parfait dishes. Pour peach mixture over graham crackers. Top with whipped topping mixture. Serves 6.

Per Serving:
calories 90
carbohydrate 16 g
protein 2 g
fat 2 g
saturated fat 1 g
cholesterol 0 mg
sodium 40 mg
fiber 3 g
soluble fiber 1 g

Watermelon Delight

½ watermelon, chilled
3 cantaloupes, chilled
3 pounds white grapes
4 pounds fresh peaches, sliced

Remove seeds from watermelon and cantaloupes and scoop out pulp with melon scoop. Add grapes and peaches and mix. Cut jagged edge around rim of watermelon half and place fruit mixture in watermelon. Makes 20 servings.

Per Serving:
calories 100
carbohydrate 23 g
protein 2 g
fat 0 g
saturated fat 0 g
cholesterol 0 mg
sodium 10 mg
fiber 4 g
soluble fiber 1 g

Apple Pie with Oatmeal Crust

Shell:
　2 cups rolled oats
　½ cup whole-wheat flour
　1 teaspoon cinnamon (to taste)
　½ teaspoon vanilla extract
　2 tablespoons canola oil
　1 tablespoon honey

Combine all ingredients and mix well; press into bottom and side of 9- to 10-inch pie pan. Mixture will be crumbly.

Filling:
　6 cups unpeeled and sliced tart apples
　　(about 6 small apples)
　1 lemon, juice and rind
　1 tablespoon honey
　2 tablespoons whole-wheat flour
　½ to 1 teaspoon cinnamon
　¼ to ½ teaspoon nutmeg
　3 egg whites
　5 ounces low-fat plain yogurt

Combine all ingredients except egg whites and yogurt; mix well and place in pie shell. Beat together egg whites and yogurt. Pour slowly over apples in shell. Bake 40 to 45 minutes at 375 degrees or until apples are soft. Serves 6.

Make several crusts and freeze for future use.

Per Serving:
calories 340
carbohydrate 58 g
protein 9 g
fat 8 g
saturated fat 1 g
cholesterol 1 mg
sodium 40 mg
fiber 8 g
soluble fiber 3 g

Emily's Applesauce Cake

1 18¼-ounce box yellow, white, or lemon cake mix
1¼ cups water
3 egg whites
⅓ cup applesauce (natural)
powdered sugar (optional)

Preheat oven to 350 degrees. Spray cake pan with nonstick spray. Blend cake mix, water, egg whites, and applesauce in a large bowl at low speed until moistened. Blend at medium speed for 2 minutes. Pour batter into pan and bake immediately. Bake for 30 to 40 minutes as directed on box; cake is done when toothpick comes out clean. Dust with powdered sugar. Cool completely in pan before cutting. Serves 12.

Variations: Serve as the cake for strawberry shortcake, or topped with any kind of fruit.

Per Serving:
calories 195
carbohydrate 35 g
protein 3 g
fat 5 g
saturated fat 1 g
cholesterol 0 mg
sodium 300 mg
fiber 1 g
soluble fiber 0 g

Easy Blueberry Crunch

4 cups fresh blueberries
1 cup firmly packed brown sugar
¾ cup all-purpose flour
¾ cup regular oats, uncooked
3 tablespoons canola oil

Spread blueberries in a 2-quart baking dish. Combine remaining ingredients, and sprinkle over blueberries. Bake at 350 degrees for 45 minutes. Serves 6.

Variations: Blackberries or other fruit may be substituted. This crunch may be microwaved on medium (60 percent) for 10 to 12 minutes instead of baking.

Per Serving:
calories 255
carbohydrate 48 g
protein 2 g
fat 6 g
saturated fat 0 g
cholesterol 0 mg
sodium 10 mg
fiber 3 g
soluble fiber 1 g

Mini-Cheesecakes

¼ cup skim milk
½ tablespoon unflavored gelatin
¼ cup (2 ounces) egg substitute
¼ cup sugar
1 cup low-fat cottage cheese
¼ teaspoon vanilla
8 vanilla wafers
fresh fruit (optional)

Per Serving:
calories 70
carbohydrate 10 g
protein 6 g
fat 1 g
saturated fat 0 g
cholesterol 4 mg
sodium 150 mg
fiber 0 g
soluble fiber 0 g

Combine milk and gelatin in 1-cup microwave measure. Beat in egg substitute and sugar. Microwave on high, uncovered, 1½ to 2 minutes or until mixture is thickened and creamy, stirring once or twice. Beat until smooth. Combine cottage cheese and vanilla in blender or food processor container and process until smooth. Blend into custard mixture. Line muffin pans with paper liners; place one vanilla wafer in bottom of each. Fill three-quarters full with cheesecake mixture. Refrigerate until set, about 2 hours. Top each with a slice of fresh fruit, if desired. Serves 8.

Variations: Substitute graham cracker crumbs for vanilla wafers. Serve with fresh or stewed fruit.

FISH, CHICKEN, MEAT, AND SEAFOOD

Dijon Fish

2 large carrots (optional)
1 cup sliced fresh mushrooms
⅓ cup sliced celery
¼ cup water
½ cup plain low-fat yogurt
1 to 2 tablespoons Dijon mustard (to taste)
4 fresh or frozen fish fillets (about 1 pound), thawed
   (choose croaker, mullet, flounder, ocean perch,
   whiting, turbot, pollack, or rockfish)
1 medium cucumber, seeded and cut lengthwise
   into 6-inch strips
1 teaspoon all-purpose flour
3 tablespoons skim milk
paprika
fresh dillweed (optional)
lemon slices, halved (optional)

Per Serving:
calories 165
carbohydrate 7 g
protein 30 g
fat 2 g
saturated fat 1 g
cholesterol 44 mg
sodium 160 mg
fiber 2 g
soluble fiber 1 g

Cut carrots into 8 long strips. In saucepan, cook carrots, mushrooms, and celery in water 5 minutes or until just tender; drain. Combine the yogurt and mustard. Brush half of yogurt mixture over one side of each fillet, reserving the rest of mixture for sauce. Lay 3 to 4 cucumber strips and 2 carrot strips crosswise on yogurt side of each fillet. Roll up fillet around vegetables. Secure with wooden picks, if necessary.

Arrange fish rolls, seam side down, in a 9 x 9 x 2-inch baking pan. Bake, uncovered, in oven at 400 degrees about 25 minutes or until fish flakes easily when tested with a fork. Remove to serving platter; remove picks.

In small saucepan stir flour into remaining yogurt mixture. Stir in milk. Add mushrooms and celery. Cook and stir over medium heat until thickened and bubbly. Spoon over fish rolls. Sprinkle with paprika. Garnish plate with fresh dillweed and lemon slices, if desired. Serves 4.

Orange Fish Fillets

1 pound orange roughy fillets
2 tablespoons frozen orange juice concentrate, thawed
1 tablespoon lemon juice
½ teaspoon dried dillweed
½ teaspoon fish seasonings
1 tablespoon finely chopped parsley
¼ cup water
2 tablespoons toasted sesame seeds

Place fish in glass casserole. Combine remaining ingredients except sesame seeds and pour over fish. Cover and marinate in refrigerator 45 minutes, turning once.

Preheat broiler. Remove fish from marinade and place on well-oiled broiler pan. Broil fish 4 inches from the heat until fish flakes, about 10 to 15 minutes. Baste often with marinade.

To serve, brush with heated marinade and top with toasted sesame seeds. Serves 4.

Per Serving:
calories 135
carbohydrate 4 g
protein 23 g
fat 3 g
saturated fat 2 g
cholesterol 42 mg
sodium 250 mg
fiber 0 g
soluble fiber 0 g

Picante Fish

1½ cups fresh mushrooms
1 medium green or red sweet pepper, seeded
    and cut into 1-inch pieces (¾ cup)
1 small onion, halved and sliced
2 tablespoons chicken broth or water
4 4-ounce fish fillets, ¾-inch thick
½ teaspoon dried oregano, crushed
1 cup picante sauce or salsa
2 tablespoons grated Parmesan cheese

Per Serving:
calories 160
carbohydrate 9 g
protein 27 g
fat 2 g
saturated fat 0 g
cholesterol 71 mg
sodium 320 mg
fiber 3 g
soluble fiber 1 g

In a 1½-quart microwave dish combine mushrooms, pepper, onion, and broth. Microwave on high 5 to 6 minutes or until tender, stirring once. In an 8 x 8 x 2-inch microwave dish, place fish fillets in an even layer. Microwave, covered, on high 5 to 6 minutes or until fish flakes easily with a fork; drain juices. With a slotted spoon, place vegetables on top of fish; sprinkle with oregano. Spoon salsa over vegetables. Microwave, uncovered, 1 to 2 minutes or until heated through. Sprinkle with Parmesan cheese. Serves 4.

Tomato Flounder

6 flounder fillets (¼ pound each)
2 small onions, sliced
2 tablespoons canola oil
1 clove garlic, finely chopped
1 16-ounce can stewed tomatoes, chopped
1 cup sliced mushrooms
¼ cup dry white wine
⅛ teaspoon basil
salt (to taste)

Per Serving:
calories 180
carbohydrate 7 g
protein 24 g
fat 6 g
saturated fat 1 g
cholesterol 42 mg
sodium 270 mg
fiber 1 g
soluble fiber 0 g

In oblong microwave dish, combine onion, oil, and garlic; microwave, covered, 3 to 3½ minutes on high. Stir in tomatoes, mushrooms, wine, and basil. Microwave, covered, 3 minutes on high. Microwave an additional 3 to 4 minutes on medium high. Arrange fish seam-side down in sauce; spoon sauce over the fish. Salt to taste. Microwave, covered, 5 to 6 minutes on high until fish is done. Let stand 5 minutes before serving. Serves 6.

Steamed Red Snapper

1 pound red snapper fillets
4 lemon slices
¾ cup chopped onion (1 small onion)
¼ cup dry white wine
1 teaspoon grated lemon rind
¼ teaspoon black pepper
2 tablespoons chopped fresh parsley

Per Serving:
calories 110
carbohydrate 3 g
protein 23 g
fat 1 g
saturated fat 0 g
cholesterol 42 mg
sodium 80 mg
fiber 1 g
soluble fiber 0 g

In a 12 x 8-inch baking dish, arrange fillets in a single layer. Top evenly with remaining ingredients. Cover loosely with waxed paper; microwave on high 4 to 7 minutes or until fish flakes easily with a fork. Serves 4.

Marinated Swordfish Steaks

2 boneless swordfish steaks (¼ pound each)
2 tablespoons orange juice
2 tablespoons reduced-sodium soy sauce
1 tablespoon lemon juice
1½ teaspoons ketchup
½ teaspoon minced and pared ginger root
½ small garlic clove, minced
¼ teaspoon cornstarch
2 lemon wedges

Per Serving:
calories 190
carbohydrate 4 g
protein 30 g
fat 6 g
saturated fat 2 g
cholesterol 56 mg
sodium 410 mg
fiber 0 g
soluble fiber 0 g

Place fish in single layer in shallow glass container; set aside. In 1-cup measure or small bowl combine orange juice, soy sauce, lemon juice, ketchup, ginger root, and garlic; pour over fish. Cover with plastic wrap and refrigerate for at least 30 minutes.

Remove swordfish from marinade and set aside. Strain marinade into a small saucepan; discard ginger and garlic. Add cornstarch to marinade and stir to dissolve; cook over medium heat, stirring frequently, until mixture is smooth and thickened, 5 to 7 minutes.

Preheat grill or broiler. Set fish on grill or on rack in broiling pan; brush with half of the marinade and grill over hot coals (or broil) for 3 to 4 minutes. Carefully turn fish over; brush with remaining marinade and cook until fish flakes easily when tested with a fork and is lightly browned, 3 to 4 minutes longer. Serve each portion with a lemon wedge. Serves 2.

Chicken à l'Orange

12 ounces chicken breast, skinned and boned
paprika
¼ cup orange juice
2 tablespoons orange marmalade
⅛ teaspoon black pepper
1 medium carrot, shredded
2 green onions, sliced (including tops)
1 tablespoon sugar
2 teaspoons cornstarch

Arrange chicken breasts in 10 x 6-inch microwave baking dish. Sprinkle with paprika. Combine juice, marmalade, and pepper. Spoon over chicken. Top with carrot and onions. Cover with plastic wrap and microwave on high 12 to 14 minutes or until chicken is done.

Drain juices into 2-cup microwave measure. Mix in sugar and cornstarch and microwave on high, uncovered, 1 to 1½ minutes or until sauce boils and thickens, stirring once. Pour sauce over chicken before serving. Serves 4.

Serve with rice and mushroom pilaf, fresh green beans, and whole-wheat rolls.

Per Serving:
calories 190
carbohydrate 14 g
protein 27 g
fat 3 g
saturated fat 1 g
cholesterol 72 mg
sodium 70 mg
fiber 1 g
soluble fiber 0 g

Light Chicken Cacciatore

1 cup onion, chopped
4 garlic cloves, minced
2 teaspoons canola oil
½ pound mushrooms, thinly sliced
1 green pepper, chopped
1 cup celery, chopped
2 16-ounce cans drained tomatoes
1 cup tomato sauce
2 bay leaves
3 teaspoons Worcestershire sauce
3 teaspoons oregano
1 teaspoon allspice
dash of black pepper
dash of cayenne pepper
18 ounces chicken breasts, skinned and boned
2 cups dry noodles

Per Serving:
calories 360
carbohydrate 42 g
protein 33 g
fat 7 g
saturated fat 1 g
cholesterol 74 mg
sodium 620 mg
fiber 6 g
soluble fiber 2 g

In a large skillet sauté onion and garlic in oil. Add mushrooms, green peppers, and celery. Sauté a few minutes longer. Add remaining ingredients except chicken and noodles; bring to boil. Add chicken, cover, reduce heat and simmer 30 minutes. Uncover and simmer an additional 20 to 30 minutes. Discard bay leaves. Prepare noodles according to package directions. Serve chicken and sauce over noodles. Serves 6.

Melt-in-Your-Mouth Chicken Kiev

3 teaspoons canola oil
4 tablespoons seasoned dry bread crumbs
3 tablespoons grated Parmesan cheese
½ teaspoon paprika
18 ounces chicken breasts, skinned and boned
salt and pepper (to taste)
6 teaspoons snipped chives

Per Serving:
calories 185
carbohydrate 4 g
protein 29 g
fat 6 g
saturated fat 2 g
cholesterol 75 mg
sodium 150 mg
fiber 0 g
soluble fiber 0 g

Combine bread crumbs, Parmesan cheese, and paprika; set aside.

Place each chicken breast half between sheets of plastic wrap. Pound with smooth side of meat mallet or rolling pin until ¼-inch thick. Sprinkle each piece with salt and pepper and 1 teaspoon chives. Spoon ½ teaspoon oil over each piece. Tuck in sides and fold over ends to form roll. Press to seal chicken surfaces together.

Roll each in crumb mixture, coating well. Place in 9-inch microwave pie plate. Refrigerate at least 30 minutes to chill. Cover with paper towel.

Microwave on high 12 to 15 minutes or until chicken is done, rotating dish twice. Serves 6.

Peach and Ginger Chicken

12 ounces chicken breasts, skinned and boned
1 8-ounce can peach slices in light syrup
1 teaspoon cornstarch
½ teaspoon grated freshginger root
   or ⅛ teaspoon ground ginger
¼ teaspoon salt
½ of an 8-ounce can sliced water chestnuts, drained
2 cups hot cooked rice
1 6-ounce package frozen pea pods, cooked and drained

Per Serving:
calories 270
carbohydrate 31 g
protein 30 g
fat 3 g
saturated fat 1 g
cholesterol 72 mg
sodium 200 mg
fiber 5 g
soluble fiber 2 g

Spray a large skillet with nonstick spray and preheat. Add chicken and cook over medium heat about 20 minutes until tender and no longer pink; turn to brown evenly. Remove from skillet; keep warm.

Meanwhile, drain peaches, reserving juice. Add water to juice to equal ½ cup. Dissolve cornstarch in 1 teaspoon cold water. Stir in cornstarch, ginger root, and salt. Add to skillet. Cook and stir until thickened and bubbly, then cook and stir 1 minute more. Gently stir in peaches and water chestnuts; heat through and then simmer for about 10 minutes.

On a serving platter or 4 individual plates, arrange rice, pea pods, and chicken. Spoon sauce over chicken. Serves 4.

Italian Chicken and Artichokes

3 tablespoons olive oil, divided
1 cup chopped onion
1 cup sliced fresh mushrooms
¼ cup chopped green pepper
½ cup chopped carrots
1 clove garlic, minced
¼ cup flour
½ teaspoon salt
½ teaspoon black pepper
1 2½- to 3-pound chicken, skinned and cut up
1 can stewed tomatoes
1 14-ounce can artichoke hearts, drained and halved
1 8-ounce can tomato sauce
½ cup dry white wine
1 teaspoon dried Italian seasoning
cooked pasta of your choice

*May also be
served over rice.*

Per Serving:
calories 390
carbohydrate 47 g
protein 31 g
fat 9 g
saturated fat 3 g
cholesterol 104 mg
sodium 420 mg
fiber 6 g
soluble fiber 2 g

In a 12-inch skillet cook onion, mushrooms, green pepper, carrot, and garlic in 1 tablespoon hot oil until tender but not brown. Remove vegetables from skillet; set aside.

In a medium bowl combine flour, ½ teaspoon salt and pepper. Add chicken pieces, a few at a time, coating all sides. Brown chicken in remaining hot oil over medium heat 10 minutes, turning occasionally (sprinkle any remaining flour mixture over chicken before browning). Return vegetables to skillet; add undrained tomatoes, artichoke hearts, tomato sauce, wine, and Italian seasoning. Heat to boiling; reduce heat and simmer, covered, 35 to 40 minutes or until chicken is tender, stirring once or twice. Transfer chicken to platter, keep warm. Boil sauce gently, uncovered, 5 minutes or until desired consistency. Serve chicken and sauce on top of cooked pasta. Serves 6.

Baked Lemon Chicken

2 tablespoons canola oil
grated peel and juice of ½ fresh lemon
24 sesame melba toast rounds, made into crumbs
1 teaspoon onion powder
1 teaspoon paprika
18 ounces chicken breasts, skinned and boned

In shallow dish combine oil, lemon peel, and juice. In separate dish, combine crumbs, onion powder, and paprika. Dip chicken into oil mixture, then roll in crumb mixture. Arrange chicken on rack in shallow baking dish; top evenly with any remaining oil or crumb mixture. Cover loosely with foil; bake at 400 degrees for 40 minutes. Remove foil; continue to bake about 20 minutes or until chicken is well browned and tender. Serves 6.

Variations: One 2½- to 3-pound chicken, cut up and skinned, may be used instead of chicken breasts.

Serve with rice, steamed vegetables, and whole-wheat rolls.

Per Serving:
calories 240
carbohydrate 12 g
protein 29 g
fat 8 g
saturated fat 1 g
cholesterol 72 mg
sodium 80 mg
fiber 0 g
soluble fiber 0 g

Mustard Chicken

18 ounces chicken breasts, skinned and boned
½ cup prepared mustard
3 tablespoons lime juice
1 tablespoon canola oil
2½ tablespoons honey
½ cup water
1 teaspoon ground coriander
2 teaspoons grated lime peel
lettuce leaves
lime wedges for garnish

Per Serving:
calories 190
carbohydrate 9 g
protein 27 g
fat 5 g
saturated fat 1 g
cholesterol 72 mg
sodium 200 mg
fiber 0 g
soluble fiber 0 g

Place chicken into shallow glass pan. Whisk together mustard, lime juice, oil, honey, water, coriander and lime peel; pour over chicken and cover. Marinate chicken 3 hours in the refrigerator, turning once or twice.

Preheat oven to 350 degrees. Place chicken pieces in ovenproof baking dish and bake for 30 minutes or until chicken is tender, basting once with remaining marinade after first 15 minutes of baking. Serve on a bed of lettuce leaves and garnish with lime wedges. Serves 6.

Sweet 'n' Sour Chicken

8 ounces uncooked linguine, broken into 2-inch lengths
1 cup sliced carrots
1 tablespoon water
12 ounces chicken breasts, skinned and boned
2 green onions, sliced (including tops)
1 clove minced garlic
1 cup sliced zucchini (about 1 medium)
½ cup sliced green pepper
1 8-ounce can pineapple chunks in unsweetened juice
water
2 tablespoons packed brown sugar
1 tablespoon cornstarch
1 tablespoon soy sauce
1 teaspoon grated fresh ginger root
1 tablespoon sliced pimiento

Cook linguine as directed on package. Drain, rinse, and set aside. Combine carrots and 1 tablespoon water in 1½-quart microwave casserole. Cover and microwave on high 2½ to 3 minutes or until just about tender.

Cut chicken into 1-inch pieces. Add to carrots; mix lightly. Add onions, garlic, zucchini, and green pepper. Microwave on high, uncovered, 5 to 6 minutes or until chicken is tender and vegetables are tender-crisp, stirring once. Set aside.

Drain juice from pineapple into 2-cup microwave measure. Add water to make 1 cup. Blend in brown sugar, cornstarch, soy sauce, and ginger until smooth. Microwave on high, uncovered, 2½ to 3½ minutes or until mixture boils and thickens, stirring once. Pour over chicken mixture. Add pineapple chunks, pimiento, and linguine; mix lightly. Cover and microwave on high 3 to 4 minutes or until heated through, stirring once. Serves 5.

This exceptionally tasty dish is lighter than traditional sweet and sour dishes.

Only bread is needed to complete this meal.

Per Serving:
calories 360
carbohydrate 54 g
protein 28 g
fat 4 g
saturated fat 1 g
cholesterol 58 mg
sodium 350 mg
fiber 5 g
soluble fiber 2 g

Homestyle Brisket

2 pounds fresh beef brisket, with all visible
   fat trimmed off
8 green onions or scallions, whole
2 medium-sized onions, peeled and quartered
8 celery stalks, cut into 3-inch pieces
8 carrots, peeled and cut into 3-inch pieces
1 bay leaf
½ teaspoon dried thyme
1 teaspoon salt
¼ teaspoon black pepper
7 cups boiling water

Per Serving:
calories 226
carbohydrate 14 g
protein 25 g
fat 7 g
saturated fat 2 g
cholesterol 69 mg
sodium 410 mg
fiber 5 g
soluble fiber 2 g

In large, heavy pot put beef and half of vegetables, bay leaf, thyme, salt, and pepper. Pour boiling water over ingredients and bring to a boil over medium heat. Cover; reduce heat to low and simmer 2½ hours. Remove cooked vegetables with a slotted spoon and set aside. Add remaining vegetables to beef. Cover pot and simmer 30 to 45 minutes longer, until vegetables and meat are tender. Using a slotted spoon, remove vegetables and meat from broth. Slice meat thin and arrange on a platter with vegetables. Serve with broth. Serves 6.

Variations: Add new potatoes for an extra vegetable.

Dijon Flank Steak

2 pounds lean flank steak, well-trimmed
⅛ cup grainy-style Dijon mustard
1 tablespoon lime juice
1 tablespoon reduced-sodium soy sauce
1 teaspoon Louisiana hot sauce
½ teaspoon Worcestershire sauce
½ teaspoon finely minced garlic
½ teaspoon finely minced fresh ginger root
freshly ground black pepper (to taste)

Per Serving:
calories 280
carbohydrate 1 g
protein 48 g
fat 9 g
saturated fat 3 g
cholesterol 122 mg
sodium 150 mg
fiber 0 g
soluble fiber 0 g

Place the steak in a large glass or ceramic dish. In a medium bowl whisk remaining ingredients together, pour over meat, coating both sides, cover, and marinate for 1 hour at room temperature or for 2 to 3 hours in the refrigerator; turn steak over once while marinating.

Preheat broiler or outdoor grill. Remove steak from marinade and broil or grill for 5 minutes on each side or until cooked to the desired doneness, basting occasionally with the marinade. Slice on bias and serve immediately. Serves 6.

Variations: Hoisin sauce (also called haisein sauce or Peking sauce) can be used instead of Louisiana hot sauce.

Tom's Marinated Round Steak

¼ cup low-salt soy sauce
2 tablespoons dry sherry
1 tablespoon honey
1 teaspoon dry mustard
½ teaspoon minced garlic
¼ teaspoon ground ginger
2 pounds beef top or bottom round steak,
   about 1½-inches thick

Mix soy sauce, sherry, honey, mustard, garlic, and ginger in large glass pan. Add steak and turn once to coat both sides. Cover and let marinate 2 hours at room temperature, turning once. Heat broiler. Place steak on broiler rack of broiling pan. For medium-rare steak broil 3 to 5 inches from heat source for 7 minutes; turn and broil 5 minutes longer. Serves 4.

*Grill outdoors
for charbroiled
flavor.*

Per Serving:
calories 425
carbohydrate 5 g
protein 72 g
fat 13 g
saturated fat 5 g
cholesterol 184 mg
sodium 430 mg
fiber 0 g
soluble fiber 0 g

Savory Steak Jardin

1 pound beef round steak, trimmed
   and tenderized
2 tablespoons margarine
1 cup chopped onions
1 11-ounce can condensed Cheddar cheese soup
¾ cup beef broth
1½ teaspoons garlic salt
¼ teaspoon black pepper
2 cups each sliced carrots and celery
1 cup sliced mushrooms
3 cups hot cooked brown rice
fresh parsley (optional)

Per Serving:
calories 365
carbohydrate 36 g
protein 30 g
fat 11 g
saturated fat 4 g
cholesterol 71 mg
sodium 480 mg
fiber 6 g
soluble fiber 1 g

continued

Cut meat into narrow strips. Brown on all sides in hot margarine. Add onions and sauté until tender-crisp. Stir in soup, broth, and seasonings. Add carrots. Cover and simmer about 20 minutes or until meat is tender. Stir in celery and mushrooms; cook 10 minutes longer. Serve over bed of rice. Garnish with fresh parsley, if desired. Serves 6.

Gingered Round Steak

**1 pound beef round steak (cut into 4 portions
    1-inch thick)**
⅔ cup water
1¼ teaspoons peeled, minced fresh ginger root
1 teaspoon seeded, chopped canned jalapeño pepper
½ teaspoon beef-flavored bouillon granules
1 small clove garlic, minced
⅛ teaspoon cracked pepper
1 tablespoon chopped fresh cilantro
    ***or* 1 teaspoon coriander**
Fresh cilantro leaves (optional)

Trim fat from steaks. Place a nonstick skillet over medium-high heat until hot. Add steaks, and cook over medium heat 5 minutes on each side or to desired degree of doneness. Remove from skillet; keep warm. Wipe drippings from skillet with paper towels. Add water, ginger root, jalapeño pepper, bouillon granules, garlic, and cracked pepper to skillet. Bring to a boil; reduce heat to medium. Cook, uncovered, 5 minutes or until reduced to ¼ cup. Stir in chopped cilantro. Spoon ginger sauce over steaks. Garnish with cilantro leaves if desired. Serves 4.

*Make sauce
ahead and reheat
to serve.*

*May be baked
instead of
prepared in a
skillet.*

Per Serving:
calories 235
carbohydrate 1 g
protein 36 g
fat 7 g
saturated fat 2 g
cholesterol 92 mg
sodium 100 mg
fiber 0 g
soluble fiber 0 g

Mustard Glazed Pork Chops

4 pork loin chops, cut ¾-inch thick
1 pound whole tiny new potatoes, sliced ¼-inch thick
½ cup water
¼ cup snipped dried apricots
2 tablespoons brown sugar
2 tablespoons vinegar
3 green onions, sliced
1 teaspoon instant chicken bouillon granules
¼ teaspoon ground turmeric
¼ teaspoon ground red pepper
2 tablespoons cold water
2 tablespoons cornstarch
¼ cup water
4 teaspoons dry mustard

The mustard glaze may be used with ham or other meat and poultry.

Per Serving:
calories 360
carbohydrate 40 g
protein 22 g
fat 11 g
saturated fat 4 g
cholesterol 63 mg
sodium 200 mg
fiber 3 g
soluble fiber 1 g

Preheat boiler. Trim fat from chops. Place chops on unheated rack of broiler pan. Broil 3 inches from heat for 12 to 14 minutes or until no pink remains, turning once halfway though cooking. Meanwhile, place potatoes in a steamer basket; sprinkle lightly with salt and pepper. Place over boiling water. Cover and steam for 10 to 12 minutes or until tender.

Mustard glaze. In a 1-quart saucepan combine apricots, brown sugar, vinegar, green onions, bouillon granules, turmeric, and red pepper with ½ cup water. Bring to boil; reduce heat, cover, and simmer 5 to 10 minutes or until apricots are tender. Stir together the 2 tablespoons cold water and cornstarch; stir into apricot mixture. Cook and stir until thickened and bubbly. Cook and stir 2 minutes more. Remove from heat. Stir together the ¼ cup water and mustard; stir into glaze; DO NOT COOK.

To serve, arrange potatoes on individual dinner plates; top each with a pork chop; spoon glaze over each chop. Serves 4.

Scallops Supreme

1 tablespoon lemon juice
2 tablespoons dry white wine
¼ teaspoon salt
⅛ teaspoon white pepper
1 pound fresh or thawed frozen scallops
2 teaspoons cornstarch
2 teaspoons canola oil
2 tablespoons dry bread crumbs
⅛ teaspoon paprika
2 tablespoons snipped parsley

Per Serving:
calories 170
carbohydrate 6 g
protein 27 g
fat 4 g
saturated fat 0 g
cholesterol 60 mg
sodium 220 mg
fiber 0 g
soluble fiber 0 g

Combine lemon juice, wine, salt, and pepper in 8-inch round microwave baking dish; blend well. Add scallops in single layer. Cover with waxed paper and microwave on high 4 to 5 minutes or until scallops are set, stirring once.

Drain juices into 1-cup microwave measure. Blend in cornstarch and microwave, uncovered, on high 45 to 60 seconds or until mixture boils and thickens, stirring once. Pour over scallops. Set aside.

Microwave oil on high in uncovered 1-cup microwave measure 30 seconds. Stir in bread crumbs and paprika. Sprinkle on scallops; top with parsley. Serves 4.

Shrimp Scampi

1 clove garlic, minced
1 teaspoon canola oil
8 ounces fresh shrimp, peeled and deveined
   or frozen uncooked large shrimp, rinsed
   and drained
½ cup fresh pea pods
2 tablespoons snipped parsley
½ teaspoon cornstarch
½ teaspoon lemon juice
dash salt
6 cherry tomatoes, halved

Per Serving:
calories 160
carbohydrate 10 g
protein 23 g
fat 3 g
saturated fat 0 g
cholesterol 170 mg
sodium 170 mg
fiber 3 g
soluble fiber 1 g

Microwave garlic and oil on high in uncovered 8-inch round microwave baking dish 1½ to 2 minutes or until tender. Mix in shrimp, pea pods, and parsley. Cover with waxed paper and microwave on high 4 to 4½ minutes or until shrimp are firm and opaque, stirring once or twice. Drain juice from shrimp into 1-cup microwave measure. Stir cornstarch, lemon juice, and salt into juice, blending well. Microwave, uncovered, on high 45 to 60 seconds or until mixture boils and thickens, stirring once. Pour mixture over shrimp; add tomatoes. Microwave, uncovered, on high 1 to 1½ minutes or until heated through. Serves 2.

Variations: Frozen pea pods may be substituted for fresh.

Tropical Shrimp Kebabs

1 8¼-ounce can pineapple chunks
   in heavy syrup
1 tablespoon canola oil
3 medium cloves garlic, crushed
⅛ teaspoon ground ginger
⅛ teaspoon ground turmeric
1 tablespoon tomato paste
½ pound fresh shrimp, peeled and deveined
½ teaspoon salt
1 tablespoon lime juice
dash hot red pepper sauce

Per Serving:
calories 245
carbohydrate 21 g
protein 22 g
fat 8 g
saturated fat 0 g
cholesterol 170 mg
sodium 330 mg
fiber 1 g
soluble fiber 0 g

Drain pineapple; reserve ¼ cup syrup. In skillet, heat oil over medium-high heat. Sauté garlic, spices, and tomato paste 2 minutes. Add shrimp; sauté 2 minutes. Stir in pineapple syrup and remaining ingredients; boil. Add pineapple; place in bowl. Accompany with picks to make kebabs. Serves 2.

MAIN DISHES

Down-Home Beans and Beef

1 tablespoon canola oil
1 cup chopped onion
1 cup chopped green pepper
½ pound lean ground beef
1 15-ounce can pinto beans, drained
1 15-ounce can butter beans, drained
1 15-ounce can great northern beans, drained
1 15-ounce can stewed tomatoes, chopped
½ teaspoon red pepper
⅛ teaspoon garlic salt
¼ teaspoon salt (optional)
2 tablespoons soy sauce (reduced salt)

Heat a 2-quart saucepan over moderate heat for 1 minute. Add oil and swirl to coat pan. Add onions and green peppers; cook and stir over moderate heat until onions are soft. Add meat and cook until meat is well browned; drain. Add remaining ingredients, heat and serve. Serves 6.

Serve over pasta or rice.

Per Serving:
calories 445
carbohydrate 61 g
protein 28 g
fat 10 g
saturated fat 3 g
cholesterol 32 mg
sodium 380 mg
fiber 16 g
soluble fiber 5 g

Jalapeño Black-Eyed Peas with Rice

½ cup uncooked long-grain rice
1 15-ounce can black-eyed peas with jalapeños, drained
½ cup chopped green onion
1 tablespoon canola oil (optional)
1 16-ounce can stewed tomatoes, diced and drained
¼ teaspoon salt
¼ teaspoon paprika
dash cayenne pepper
dash black pepper

Prepare rice as directed. Stir in remaining ingredients; cover. Microwave on high 3 minutes, stirring once. Serves 4.

Variations: For an extra-spicy dish, substitute a can of stewed tomatoes with garlic, cumin, and jalapeños (Mexican-style) for tomatoes and leave out the paprika, cayenne, and pepper.

Serve with asparagus, broccoli, or green beans.

Per Serving:
calories 300
carbohydrate 53 g
protein 12 g
fat 5 g
saturated fat 0 g
cholesterol 0 mg
sodium 560 mg
fiber 13 g
soluble fiber 5 g

Nancy's Five Bean Dinner

1 15- to 16-ounce can kidney beans
1 15- to 16-ounce can chick peas (garbanzo beans)
1 15- to 16-ounce can great northern beans
1 15- to 16-ounce can red beans
1 15- to 16-ounce can pork and beans
1 pound lean ground beef, browned and drained
1 15- to 16-ounce can tomatoes (including juice)
   or 2 to 3 fresh tomatoes, chopped
1 chopped onion
½ cup vinegar
½ cup brown sugar

Per Serving:
calories 395
carbohydrate 52 g
protein 25 g
fat 10 g
saturated fat 3 g
cholesterol 39 mg
sodium 680 mg
fiber 17 g
soluble fiber 7 g

Drain all beans except the pork and beans. Pour all ingredients in a crockpot and cook 8 hours on low heat. Serves 10.

Ground beef can be browned in the microwave to save time.

Taco Salad

1 16-ounce can chili hot beans, drained
½ can (7- to 8-ounce) stewed tomatoes, Mexican-style, drained
½ cup chopped onion
4 tablespoons salsa
4 corn tortillas, toasted
½ cup (2 ounces) reduced-calorie Cheddar cheese, shredded
4 large black olives, sliced (optional)
salsa (to taste)

Mix beans, tomatoes, onions, and salsa. Place tortillas on four salad plates. Spoon mixture over tortillas. Sprinkle cheese over top. Top with sliced black olives if desired. Serves 4.

Variations: Use low-sodium canned tomatoes and beans to reduce sodium content. Flavor as desired with salsa or green chilies.

This tasty salad can be served on lettuce or as a side dish for a Mexican dinner.

Per Serving:
calories 260
carbohydrates 40 g
protein 14 g
fat 5 g
saturated fat 2 g
cholesterol 8 mg
sodium 750 mg
fiber 9 g
soluble fiber 4 g

Fast Hoppin' John

2 cups cooked rice
1 tablespoon canola oil
¼ pound turkey ham, coarsely chopped
½ cup chopped onion
1 garlic clove, minced
1 15- to 16-ounce can black-eyed peas
¼ teaspoon hot pepper sauce (to taste)
⅛ teaspoon black pepper
pinch of crushed red pepper flakes

Heat oil in nonstick skillet. Stir in ham, onion, and garlic and brown until onion is tender. Stir in peas, rice, hot pepper sauce, pepper, and pepper flakes; cook on low to medium for 5 minutes until thoroughly heated. Serves 4.

Per Serving:
calories 310
carbohydrate 47 g
protein 17 g
fat 6 g
saturated fat 1 g
cholesterol 16 mg
sodium 300 mg
fiber 12 g
soluble fiber 5 g

Rapid Rice and Black Bean Meal

¾ cup uncooked long-grain brown rice
1 10-ounce package frozen corn kernels
1 15- to 16-ounce can black beans, rinsed and drained
½ cup chopped green pepper
¼ teaspoon salt (to taste)
½ cup salsa
¼ cup light sour cream
½ cup (2 ounces) shredded reduced-fat Cheddar cheese

Cook rice according to package directions, adding corn to rice during the last five minutes of cooking; cool. Mix rice, corn, black beans, green pepper, and salt in a large serving bowl. Top each serving with 2 tablespoons salsa, 1 teaspoon sour cream, and 2 tablespoons shredded cheese. Serves 4.

Serve with bread and you have a meal.

Per Serving:
calories 450
carbohydrate 85 g
protein 23 g
fat 9 g
saturated fat 2 g
cholesterol 15 mg
sodium 640 mg
fiber 12 g
soluble fiber 4 g

Chicken-Broccoli Bake with Rice

1 cup uncooked long-grain rice
¼ cup (2 ounces) egg substitute
¼ cup grated Parmesan cheese
½ cup fine dry bread crumbs
¼ teaspoon paprika
12 ounces chicken breasts, skinned and boned
1 medium head broccoli, cut into 2-inch pieces
   (about 4 cups)

Sauce (optional):
2 teaspoons canola oil
1 tablespoon all-purpose flour
⅔ cup skim milk
¼ teaspoon salt (to taste)
¼ cup (1 ounce) grated Cheddar cheese

*Buy precut
broccoli at a
salad bar.*

Per Serving:
calories 440
carbohydrate 56 g
protein 40 g
fat 6 g
saturated fat 2 g
cholesterol 77 mg
sodium 320 mg
fiber 4 g
soluble fiber 2 g

In 12 x 8 x 2-inch microwave baking dish combine rice and 2¼ cups water; spread rice in even layer. Cover with plastic wrap, folding back one corner to allow excess steam to escape; cook on high 9 minutes.

Meanwhile, lightly beat egg substitute in shallow dish. In separate dish combine Parmesan cheese, bread crumbs, and paprika. One at a time, dip chicken pieces in egg substitute, then in crumb mixture to coat well.

Remove baking dish from microwave. Arrange chicken over rice in center of dish. Arrange broccoli pieces over rice at each end of the dish, placing pieces so flower ends point toward center. Sprinkle chicken with any remaining crumb mixture. Cover dish with plastic wrap, folding back one corner, and microwave on high 9 to 11 minutes until broccoli is tender and chicken is done. Set aside. *continued*

To serve, rearrange broccoli so stems point toward center. Pour half of sauce over broccoli; sprinkle with paprika, if desired. Serve remaining sauce on the side. Serves 4.

Sauce preparation: Combine oil and flour in a 2-cup microwave dish and heat, uncovered, on high 30 seconds. Gradually stir in milk to blend well; add salt. Cook, uncovered, on high 2 to 2½ minutes until mixture boils and thickens, stirring once. Stir in Cheddar cheese until melted.

All the sauce may be served on the side. The dish also tastes fine without the sauce and contains fewer calories.

Chicken Cacciatore
and Green Beans

1 teaspoon canola oil
¼ cup chopped onion
¼ cup chopped green pepper
1 garlic clove, minced
8 ounces chicken breast, skinned and boned,
    cut into 1-inch cubes
½ cup canned tomatoes, drained and chopped
½ cup frozen cut green beans
¼ teaspoon oregano leaves
⅛ teaspoon salt

Serve over rice or noodles.

Per Serving:
calories 260
carbohydrate 12 g
protein 37 g
fat 7 g
saturated fat 1 g
cholesterol 96 mg
sodium 400 mg
fiber 4 g
soluble fiber 1 g

In 8- or 10-inch skillet heat oil over medium heat; add onion, green pepper, and garlic and sauté for 2 minutes. Add chicken to skillet and continue to sauté until chicken is no longer pink, about 5 minutes. Stir in tomatoes, green beans, and seasonings. Reduce heat to low and let simmer, stirring occasionally, for 5 to 8 minutes until chicken is cooked through and tender. Serves 2.

Variations: Use fresh or canned green beans.

Jambalaya in a Hurry

2 teaspoons olive or canola oil
1 small sweet green pepper, cored, seeded and chopped
1 medium-sized stalk celery, thinly sliced
1 small yellow onion, chopped
2 cloves garlic, minced
1 16-ounce can low-sodium tomatoes, chopped,
    with their juice
½ cup low-sodium chicken broth
¼ teaspoon dried thyme, crumbled
¼ teaspoon crushed red pepper
⅛ teaspoon ground allspice
⅛ teaspoon cloves
⅛ teaspoon cayenne pepper
12 ounces chicken breast, skinned and boned,
    cooked and cubed
½ pound raw small shrimp, shelled and deveined
2 cups cooked long-grain brown or white rice

Per Serving:
calories 385
carbohydrate 38 g
protein 42 g
fat 7 g
saturated fat 1 g
cholesterol 157 mg
sodium 310 mg
fiber 5 g
soluble fiber 1 g

Heat oil in a large saucepan over medium heat for 1 minute.
Add green pepper, celery, onion, and garlic and sauté, stirring frequently, about 5 minutes or until onion is soft.

Add the tomatoes, chicken broth, thyme, red pepper, allspice,
cloves, and cayenne pepper. Bring to a boil then reduce heat
and simmer, uncovered, for 15 minutes. Add chicken, shrimp,
and rice; cook 5 minutes longer, stirring frequently, until
shrimp are pink. Serves 4.

Kathy's Seafood Pasta Delight

12 ounces uncooked rainbow twirls
1 bell pepper, chopped
1 small onion, chopped
10 ounces sliced mushrooms
2 tomatoes or cherry tomatoes, chopped
1½ ounces pitted black olives, sliced
¼ cup grated Parmesan cheese
1 cup chopped celery
1 8-ounce bottle no-oil Italian dressing
1 pound imitation crabmeat flakes

Cook rainbow twirls according to package directions; drain. Add remaining ingredients to pasta and mix well. Refrigerate until ready to serve. Serves 6.

*May be made
ahead and
refrigerated for
up to 48 hours.*

Per Serving:
calories 260
carbohydrate 39 g
protein 15 g
fat 5 g
saturated fat 2 g
cholesterol 34 mg
sodium 700 mg
fiber 4 g
soluble fiber 1 g

Classic Tuna Noodle Casserole

1 8-ounce package wide egg noodles
1 tablespoon canola oil
¼ pound mushrooms, sliced
1 cup chopped onion
½ cup chopped green pepper
⅓ cup chopped celery
3 teaspoons all-purpose wheat flour
2 cups skim milk
1 cup chicken broth
¼ teaspoon salt
¼ teaspoon black pepper
2 6½-ounce cans tuna in spring water, drained

Per Serving:
calories 285
carbohydrate 35 g
protein 26 g
fat 5 g
saturated fat 1 g
cholesterol 71 mg
sodium 460 mg
fiber 3 g
soluble fiber 1 g

Preheat oven to 350 degrees. Coat a 2-quart casserole dish with nonstick spray. In saucepan cook noodles according to package directions until done.

In medium skillet melt oil over medium heat. Add mushrooms, onion, green pepper, and celery. Sauté about 5 minutes, stirring occasionally. Stir in flour until smooth; cook, stirring frequently, about 5 minutes. Gradually add milk and chicken broth, stirring until smooth. Add salt and pepper. Simmer 10 minutes, stirring occasionally.

In large bowl combine noodles, sauce, and tuna; toss well. Spoon into prepared casserole and bake 30 minutes. Let stand 10 minutes before serving. Serves 6.

Variations: May be microwaved on medium for 20 minutes. Substitute carrots for celery for more color.

Macaroni and Cheese Surprise

6 cups hot water
¼ teaspoon salt
1 cup rotini or regular macaroni
3 medium carrots, sliced
2 tablespoons chopped onion
2 tablespoons chopped celery
2 tablespoons water
2 cups broccoli pieces
⅓ cup skim milk
2 teaspoons cornstarch
dash black pepper
4 ounces cubed processed cheese spread
    (about ¾ cup)

Per Serving:
calories 320
carbohydrate 46 g
protein 16 g
fat 9 g
saturated fat 3 g
cholesterol 22 mg
sodium 670 mg
fiber 6 g
soluble fiber 2 g

Combine 6 cups hot water, salt, and rotini in 2-quart microwave bowl. Microwave, uncovered, on high 12 to 14 minutes or until rotini is just about tender, stirring once. Let stand about 5 minutes. Drain and set aside.

Combine carrots, onion, celery and 2 tablespoons water in 1-quart microwave casserole; cover and microwave on high 3 minutes. Stir in broccoli; cover and microwave on high 2 to 3 minutes or until just about tender. Add milk and cornstarch; mix lightly. Add pepper and cheese spread. Cover and microwave on high 3 to 4 minutes or until sauce boils and thickens slightly, stirring once. Add rotini; mix lightly. Serves 2 to 3.

Variations: Other garden vegetables may be substituted. Mixed vegetables, green beans, or peas would be good.

Jim's Bean Burritos

1 large onion, chopped
1 8-ounce can Mexican-style stewed tomatoes, chopped
2 15¾-ounce cans chili hot beans, mashed
8 10-inch flour tortillas
½ cup bottled taco sauce
4 ounces shredded Cheddar cheese
1 cup taco sauce or salsa (optional)

Place chopped onions in 1-quart casserole dish and drain juice from tomatoes into dish. Microwave on high for 4 minutes, until tender, stirring once. Add mashed beans and chopped tomatoes and mix. Microwave on high for 1 minute. Spoon ⅛ of mixture onto edge of tortilla, spread 1 tablespoon of taco sauce over beans and sprinkle cheese on top; roll up and put in casserole dish. Arrange 8 burritos in casserole dish and microwave for 3 to 4 minutes until cheese is melted and burrito thoroughly warmed. Serve with additional taco sauce or salsa on top. Makes 8 burritos.

Per Burrito:
calories 275
carbohydrate 40 g
protein 13 g
fat 7 g
saturated fat 3 g
cholesterol 15 mg
sodium 580 mg
fiber 8 g
soluble fiber 3 g

Enchilada Stack Up

¾ **pound ground turkey**
½ **cup chopped onion**
1 8-ounce can tomato sauce
2 teaspoons chopped green chilies
1½ teaspoons chili powder
⅛ **teaspoon black pepper**
1 17-ounce can red kidney beans, drained
½ **cup sliced pitted black olives**
4 corn or flour tortillas
½ **cup (2 ounces) shredded low-fat mozzarella cheese**
¾ **cup tomato juice**

*Serve with corn
or green beans
on the side.*

Per Serving:
calories 310
carbohydrate 32 g
protein 23 g
fat 10 g
saturated fat 6 g
cholesterol 55 mg
sodium 770 mg
fiber 10 g
soluble fiber 5 g

In skillet, cook turkey and onion until meat is browned and onion is tender. Drain off excess fat. Add tomato sauce, chilies, chili powder, and pepper. Stir in drained beans and olives. Place ¼ of the meat mixture in bottom of crockery cooker; top with one tortilla and sprinkle with ¼ cup cheese. Repeat layers with meat, tortillas, and cheese. Pour tomato juice around edge of stack-up. Cover; cook on low heat setting for 5 to 6 hours or on high setting 2½ hours. Cut into wedges to serve. Carefully lift out of cooker. Serves 4.

Variations: Fresh or canned chicken may be substituted for turkey.

Crowd-Pleasing Black-Bean Enchiladas

1 large onion, chopped
1 tablespoon garlic, minced
2 teaspoons chili powder
2 teaspoons cumin
¼ teaspoon oregano
¼ teaspoon salt
⅛ teaspoon ground red pepper
2 14-ounce cans tomatoes, chopped
2 15-ounce cans black beans, drained and rinsed
12 7-inch flour tortillas
1½ cups (6 ounces) shredded Monterey Jack cheese
1 4-ounce can green chilies, drained and chopped
2 green onions, chopped
2 tablespoons chopped fresh cilantro or parsley

Serve with a side salad and Spanish rice.

Per Serving:
calories 460
carbohydrate 66 g
protein 20 g
fat 13 g
saturated fat 6 g
cholesterol 26 mg
sodium 750 mg
fiber 6 g
soluble fiber 2 g

Combine onion and garlic in medium microwave bowl. Cover with waxed paper, turning back one edge to vent. Microwave on high for 2 minutes. Stir in chili powder, cumin, oregano, salt, and red pepper. Cover and microwave 1 minute. Stir in tomatoes; microwave, uncovered, for 3 more minutes. Transfer 1 cup of tomato mixture to another bowl and reserve for topping. Add beans to remaining tomatoes and toss to combine.

For each enchilada, sprinkle about one-eighth of the cheese down center of 1 tortilla. Top with 1 heaping tablespoon green chilies and ½ cup black-bean mixture. Roll up and place seam side down in 13 x 9-inch microwave casserole. Repeat with remaining tortillas and filling. Spoon remaining tomato mixture over enchiladas. Cover and microwave 4 minutes, turning dish once at halfway, until heated through. Sprinkle with green onions and cilantro. Serves 6.

Variations: Vary the spiciness to suit your taste by using hot green chilies or milder red chilies.

Tex-Mex Frijoles

1 16-ounce can pinto beans with sauce
2 slices turkey bacon, chopped
1 tablespoon jalapeño pepper, diced
½ cup chopped onions
1 teaspoon minced garlic
½ teaspoon salt
⅓ cup flat beer or water
¼ cup chopped parsley

Add beans and sauce to large saucepan. Add bacon, jalapeños, onions, garlic, salt, and beer or water. Simmer, covered, until liquid is thickened, about 15 to 20 minutes. Stir
in parsley and serve hot. Makes 4 servings.

*May also be
prepared in the
microwave.*

Per Serving:
calories 200
carbohydrate 37 g
protein 11 g
fat 1 g
saturated fat 0 g
cholesterol 9 mg
sodium 280 mg
fiber 8 g
soluble fiber 3 g

Salsa in a Flash

1 cup chopped tomato
⅓ cup chopped green pepper
2 tablespoons minced jalapeño pepper
½ teaspoon chili powder
¼ teaspoon dried garlic chips
⅛ teaspoon salt
⅛ teaspoon black pepper

Combine first three ingredients. Add next four ingredients
and mix. Chill. Makes 20 1-tablespoon servings.

Variations: Chopped onions or chopped green onions may
be substituted for green pepper. Canned or fresh green chilies may be substituted for the jalapeño peppers.

Per Serving:
calories 6
carbohydrate 1 g
protein 0 g
fat 0 g
saturated fat 0 g
cholesterol 0 mg
sodium 40 mg
fiber 0 g
soluble fiber 0 g

Spinach Chicken Tacos

¼ cup chopped green pepper
8 ounces chicken breasts, skinned and
    boned, cooked and cubed
½ cup taco sauce
8 taco shells
2 cups chopped fresh spinach
1 small tomato, chopped
¼ cup (1 ounce) shredded reduced-calorie
    Cheddar cheese
¼ cup chopped ripe olives (optional)

Per Serving:
calories 120
carbohydrate 9 g
protein 12 g
fat 4 g
saturated fat 1 g
cholesterol 23 mg
sodium 280 mg
fiber 2 g
soluble fiber 1 g

Place green pepper in 1-quart microwave casserole. Cover and microwave on high 1 to 1½ minutes or until tender-crisp. Stir in chicken and taco sauce. Cover and microwave on high 3 to 3½ minutes or until heated through.

To serve, spoon about ¼ cup chicken mixture into each taco shell. Top each with ¼ cup spinach, 1 tablespoon each tomato and cheese, and ½ tablespoon olives. Makes 8 tacos.

Variations: Lettuce may be substituted for spinach.

Oriental Seafood Stir-Fry

1 8-ounce package imitation crabmeat flakes
  (e.g., Crab Delights)
1 10-ounce package frozen Chinese-style
  vegetables with seasoning
⅛ teaspoon garlic powder
⅛ teaspoon ground ginger
4 cups cooked rice
soy sauce, optional

Combine crabmeat flakes, vegetables with seasoning, garlic, and ginger. Heat according to directions on vegetable package. Stir and serve. Season with soy sauce, if desired. Serves 3.

Comments: Imitation crabmeat is a blend of steam-baked fish with artificial crab flavor.

Use low-salt vegetables to reduce sodium content.

Per Serving:
calories 340
carbohydrate 67 g
protein 15 g
fat 1 g
saturated fat 0 g
cholesterol 14 mg
sodium 700 mg
fiber 2 g
soluble fiber 1 g

Oriental Surprise

1 cup uncooked quick-cooking rice
½ cup reduced-calorie apricot preserves
1 tablespoon reduced-sodium soy sauce
½ teaspoon grated fresh ginger root
⅛ teaspoon crushed red pepper
1 cup sliced fresh mushrooms
1 medium green pepper, cut into strips
1 medium sweet red pepper, cut into strips
4 green onions, bias-sliced into 1-inch pieces
2 tablespoons red wine vinegar
2 tablespoons cornstarch
8 ounces chicken breasts, cooked and
    torn into strips

Per Serving:
calories 275
carbohydrate 42 g
protein 22 g
fat 2 g
saturated fat 1 g
cholesterol 48 mg
sodium 400 mg
fiber 6 g
soluble fiber 2 g

Cook rice as directed, omitting margarine and salt.

For sauce, stir together preserves, soy sauce, ginger root, and crushed red pepper; set aside.

In a 1½-quart casserole, place mushrooms, green and red pepper strips, and green onions. Pour sauce mixture over the vegetables. Toss gently until mixed. Cover and microwave on high 4 to 5 minutes or until pepper strips are tender-crisp, stirring every minute.

Stir together vinegar and cornstarch, then add mixture to casserole. Stir in chicken. Microwave, uncovered, on high for 3 to 4 minutes or until mixture is thickened and bubbly, stirring after every minute. Serves 4.

Chicken Lo Mein

1 tablespoon dark sesame or canola oil
12 ounces chicken breasts, skinned and boned,
    cut into strips
1 14-ounce can chicken broth
1 cup water
1 tablespoon minced fresh ginger root
⅛ teaspoon crushed red pepper flakes
3 tablespoons teriyaki sauce
1 large clove garlic, minced
1 8-ounce package spaghetti
1 16-ounce package frozen mixed vegetables
    containing broccoli, carrots, red peppers,
    and water chestnuts
2 green onions, sliced

Heat oil in skillet over medium-high heat. Brown chicken about 3 minutes; remove to plate. In same pan, bring broth, water, ginger, pepper flakes, teriyaki sauce, and garlic to boiling; add spaghetti. Simmer, covered, 8 minutes, stirring often. Stir in vegetables and chicken. Bring to boiling, then reduce heat and simmer, covered, another 4 minutes. Stir in onions. Serves 4.

Serve with crusty French bread.

Per Serving:
calories 500
carbohydrate 65 g
protein 41 g
fat 9 g
saturated fat 1 g
cholesterol 73 mg
sodium 690 mg
fiber 3 g
soluble fiber 1 g

Pinto Bean Chow Mein

2 tablespoons canola oil
1 cup thin-sliced carrots
1½ cups thin bias-cut celery slices
½ cup chopped onions
½ pound sliced mushrooms
1 tablespoon cornstarch
1½ cups cold water
¼ cup low-sodium soy sauce
1 15-ounce can pinto beans, drained
1 15-ounce can bean sprouts, drained
1 8-ounce can sliced water chestnuts, drained
1 8-ounce can bamboo shoots, drained

Stir-fry carrots, celery, onions, and mushrooms in oil until tender-crisp. Blend cornstarch, water, and soy sauce until smooth then stir into vegetables. Add the remaining ingredients. Cook and stir until thickened. Serve over hot brown rice or chow mein noodles. Serves 4.

Per Serving:
calories 350
carbohydrate 56 g
protein 16 g
fat 7 g
saturated fat 1 g
cholesterol 0 mg
sodium 600 mg
fiber 12 g
soluble fiber 4 g

Party Red Bean Lasagna

1 large onion, chopped
2 medium carrots, chopped
1 clove garlic, minced
1 tablespoon canola oil
1 16-ounce can tomatoes, cut up, undrained
6 ounces tomato sauce
1 16-ounce can red kidney beans, drained
1 teaspoon sugar
¼ cup snipped parsley *and* 3 tablespoons parsley
1 teaspoon dried oregano, crushed
1 teaspoon dried basil, crushed
2 cups sliced fresh mushrooms
10 ounces frozen spinach, thawed
¼ cup (2 ounces) egg substitute
1½ cups (6 ounces) shredded mozzarella cheese
1½ cups low-fat cottage cheese, drained
¼ cup grated Parmesan cheese
9 lasagna noodles, cooked

Per Serving:
calories 315
carbohydrate 38 g
protein 21 g
fat 9 g
saturated fat 4 g
cholesterol 35 mg
sodium 35 mg
fiber 7 g
soluble fiber 3 g

Cook onion, carrot, and garlic in oil. Add undrained tomatoes, tomato sauce, beans, sugar, ¼ cup parsley, oregano, basil, and 1 teaspoon salt. Bring to boil; reduce heat, cover, and simmer 15 minutes. Mash beans slightly. Add mushrooms and spinach; simmer, uncovered, 15 minutes more. Combine egg substitute, half of the mozzarella cheese, all the cottage cheese and Parmesan cheese, and 3 tablespoons parsley in a separate bowl.

Spread ½ cup bean mixture in a 13 x 9 x 2-inch dish. Arrange three noodles on top. Spread with one-third of the cheese mixture, then one-third of the remaining bean mixture. Repeat the layers twice. Bake, covered, in a 375 degree oven for 40 minutes. Top with the remaining mozzarella cheese. Bake 5 minutes more uncovered. Serves 8.

Stuffed Manicotti

1 8-ounce package manicotti shells
1 10-ounce package frozen chopped spinach
8 ounces firm tofu
¼ cup grated Parmesan cheese
1 cup fresh mushrooms, sliced
¼ cup (2 ounces) egg substitute
1 cup (4 ounces) shredded mozzarella cheese
1 28-ounce jar (4 cups) low-fat, low-sodium
    spaghetti sauce

Per Serving:
calories 470
carbohydrate 59 g
protein 25 g
fat 15 g
saturated fat 4 g
cholesterol 30 mg
sodium 750 mg
fiber 3 g
soluble fiber 1 g

Cook manicotti shells according to package directions. Drain and rinse shells with cold water; set aside.

Place spinach box on plate and microwave on high until tender (5 to 6 minutes). Combine spinach, tofu, Parmesan cheese, mushrooms, egg substitute, and half of the mozzarella cheese in small mixing bowl. Stir until well combined. Stuff spinach mixture in manicotti shells. Place half of the shells in 1-quart dish, top with half of the sauce; cover. Place remaining shells in another 1-quart dish and top with remaining sauce. Freeze one casserole dish of manicotti if desired.

Microwave one dish at high until heated through (8 to 10 minutes). Top with remaining mozzarella cheese; microwave on high until cheese is melted (about 4½ minutes). To serve frozen manicotti, thaw completely and follow above directions. Serves 4.

Variations: You may substitute other summer vegetables such as yellow squash or zucchini for spinach.

Spicy Pasta with Broccoli

1 large bunch broccoli
1 sweet yellow pepper, thinly sliced
1 medium onion, chopped
2 cloves garlic, minced
6 black olives, finely chopped
1 tablespoon currants
1 tablespoon minced fresh oregano *or*
   1 teaspoon dried oregano
1 tablespoon minced fresh parsley
⅛ teaspoon ground black pepper
1 pound linguine, uncooked
crushed red pepper (optional)

Per Serving:
calories 335
carbohydrate 68 g
protein 11 g
fat 3 g
saturated fat 0 g
cholesterol 0 mg
sodium 100 mg
fiber 5 g
soluble fiber 2 g

Trim broccoli and break into florets. Bring a large pot of water to a boil; add broccoli and cook for 10 minutes. Remove with a slotted spoon. Reserve cooking water.

Heat a large nonstick frying pan over medium heat. Add yellow pepper, onion, and garlic. Sauté, stirring, until onion and garlic are golden, about 5 to 7 minutes. Add broccoli, 1 cup of reserved cooking water, olives, currants, oregano, parsley, and black pepper. Simmer 7 to 10 minutes.

Meanwhile, bring reserved water back to a boil. Add linguine and cook until just tender; drain. In a large shallow bowl, toss the pasta with the broccoli mixture. Sprinkle with crushed red pepper. Serve immediately. Serves 6.

Linguine Primavera

1 pound linguine, cooked in unsalted water
   and drained
2 cups coarsely chopped broccoli
1 cup julienne carrot strips
1 medium onion, cut into wedges
1 teaspoon Italian seasoning
2 cloves garlic, crushed
¼ teaspoon ground black pepper
2 tablespoons canola oil
1 large tomato *or* 8 ounces canned tomatoes,
   coarsely chopped
1 cup (8 ounces) egg substitute
¼ cup grated Parmesan cheese

Per Serving:
calories 380
carbohydrate 66 g
protein 19 g
fat 5 g
saturated fat 1 g
cholesterol 4 mg
sodium 170 mg
fiber 5 g
soluble fiber 2 g

In skillet over medium heat, cook broccoli, carrots, onion, Italian seasoning, garlic, and pepper in oil for 3 minutes, stirring occasionally. Add tomato; cook for 1 minute more or until vegetables are tender-crisp. Toss with hot linguine, egg substitute, and cheese. Garnish and serve immediately. Serves 6.

Baked Rigatoni and Cheese

¼ pound uncooked rigatoni
½ cup part-skim ricotta cheese
½ cup diced part-skim mozzarella cheese
1 tablespoon grated Parmesan cheese
⅛ teaspoon freshly ground black pepper
1 cup meatless spaghetti sauce

Cook rigatoni according to directions. Combine ricotta, mozzarella, and Parmesan cheeses. Add pepper and set aside.

Spoon ½ cup sauce into a small, flat baking dish. Top with half of the cooked rigatoni. Spread cheese mixture over rigatoni. Make a layer of the remaining rigatoni and top it with the remaining sauce. Bake at 350 degrees for 20 minutes. Serves 2.

Comments: This tasty pasta recipe may be doubled and frozen or reheated for lunch.

Serve with quick garlic rolls.

Per Serving:
calories 475
carbohydrate 71 g
protein 16 g
fat 14 g
saturated fat 6 g
cholesterol 38 mg
sodium 750 mg
fiber 3 g
soluble fiber 2 g

Spinach Stuffed Shells

24 uncooked jumbo macaroni shells
1 small onion, diced
2 14½-ounce cans whole tomatoes (no added salt),
    undrained and chopped
1 6-ounce can tomato paste (no added salt)
1 8-ounce can tomato sauce (no added salt)
1 tablespoon brown sugar
½ teaspoon salt
¼ teaspoon black pepper
1 tablespoon dried oregano
2 10-ounce packages frozen chopped spinach,
    thawed and drained
1 16-ounce container 1 percent low-fat cottage cheese
1 cup (4 ounces) shredded 40 percent less fat
    mozzarella cheese
¼ teaspoon black pepper

Per Serving:
calories 212
carbohydrate 28 g
protein 17 g
fat 4 g
saturated fat 2 g
cholesterol 11 mg
sodium 665 mg
fiber 4 g
soluble fiber 1 g

Cook shells according to package directions, omitting salt; drain.

Preheat a large saucepan over medium heat; coat with non-stick cooking spray, add onion and sauté until tender. Add tomatoes and next 6 ingredients; stir well. Bring to boil, cover, reduce heat, and simmer 20 minutes, stirring occasionally.

Drain spinach; press between layers of paper towels. Combine spinach, cottage cheese, mozzarella cheese, and pepper; stir well. Fill each shell with 2 tablespoons spinach mixture.

Spoon ¼ cup sauce into each of 8 oven or microwave containers. Place 3 filled shells in each container and top with

continued

¼ cup sauce. Cover with heavy-duty plastic wrap, removing as much air as possible. Then cover with heavy-duty aluminum foil and freeze. Serves 8.

To heat frozen shells in oven, remove foil and plastic wrap, and recover dish with foil. Bake at 350 degrees for 1 hour and 10 minutes or until heated.

To heat frozen shells in microwave, remove foil and vent plastic wrap on one side. Microwave on high 5 to 7 minutes or until heated, rotating dish a half-turn after 2½ to 3½ minutes.

Tortellini Salad

4 cups hot water
½ 9-ounce package dried tortellini
    with cheese filling
1½ cups small broccoli pieces
1½ cups small cauliflower pieces
2 teaspoons olive or canola oil
2 tablespoons lemon juice
½ teaspoon Worcestershire sauce
¼ teaspoon dry mustard
¼ teaspoon dried tarragon leaves
¼ teaspoon salt
1 clove garlic, minced
2 green onions, sliced
2 tablespoons diced red pepper

Per Serving:
calories 160
carbohydrate 21 g
protein 7 g
fat 5 g
saturated fat 1 g
cholesterol 15 mg
sodium 250 mg
fiber 4 g
soluble fiber 2 g

Combine water, ½ teaspoon salt, ½ teaspoon oil, and tortellini in 2-quart microwave casserole. Microwave, uncovered, on high 13 to 15 minutes or until pasta is tender, stirring once. Drain, rinse, and set aside.

Place broccoli and cauliflower in 1½-quart shallow microwave baking dish. Cover and microwave on high 3 to 3½ minutes or until vegetables are tender-crisp. Uncover and set aside.

Combine drained tortellini and remaining ingredients in serving bowl. Add broccoli and cauliflower. Refrigerate until chilled. Serves 4.

Variations: Other vegetables such as asparagus or zucchini may be substituted for broccoli or cauliflower.

To save time, chop vegetables ahead and use precooked tortellini.

Vegetarian Spaghetti

1 large onion, thinly sliced
10 mushrooms, sliced
1 green pepper, thinly sliced
1 16-ounce package firm tofu, cut into small cubes
8 dark green olives, thinly sliced
1 15½-ounce jar low-fat spaghetti sauce
6 servings cooked spaghetti noodles

Sauté sliced onions, mushrooms, and green peppers in a skillet sprayed with nonstick cooking spray. Add tofu, then spaghetti sauce. When the mixture is warm, pour over hot cooked spaghetti. Serves 6.

Per Serving:
calories 350
carbohydrate 60 g
protein 15 g
fat 6 g
saturated fat 1 g
cholesterol 1 mg
sodium 380 mg
fiber 4 g
soluble fiber 1 g

VEGETABLES

Hot Spiced Beets

1 16-ounce can sliced beets
4 tablespoons apple cider vinegar
⅛ teaspoon allspice
⅛ teaspoon ground black pepper

Drain beets. Mix remaining ingredients in stovetop pan. Heat on medium for 5 minutes. Serve warm. Serves 4.

Variations: May be prepared in the microwave.

Per Serving:
calories 40
carbohydrate 9 g
protein 1 g
fat 0 g
saturated fat 0 g
cholesterol 0 mg
sodium 320 mg
fiber 3 g
soluble fiber 1 g

Sweet and Sour Beets

2 tablespoons thawed frozen concentrated
    orange juice
1 tablespoon lemon juice
¼ teaspoon black pepper
1 tablespoon dark brown sugar
¼ teaspoon grated orange peel
¼ teaspoon grated lemon peel
1 teaspoon canola oil
½ cup diced onions
1 16-ounce can sliced beets, drained

Per Serving:
calories 70
carbohydrate 15 g
protein 1 g
fat 1 g
saturated fat 0 g
cholesterol 0 mg
sodium 280 mg
fiber 4 g
soluble fiber 1 g

In a small bowl combine orange juice, lemon juice, salt, pepper, sugar, and orange and lemon peels. In 2-quart saucepan heat oil until bubbly hot; add onion and sauté until slightly brown. Add remaining ingredients to saucepan and bring to a boil, stirring constantly. Reduce heat and let simmer for 3 to 4 minutes to allow flavors to blend. Serves 4.

May also be prepared in the microwave.

Broccoli, Cauliflower, and Mushroom Medley

1 bunch fresh broccoli, about 1 pound	½ pound fresh mushrooms
1 head cauliflower, about 1 pound	1 tablespoon canola oil
¼ teaspoon salt	½ teaspoon dried marjoram leaves
dash of black pepper	1 tablespoon lemon juice
2 tablespoons water	1 slice lemon, twisted (optional)

Sprinkle cooked vegetables with natural butter-flavored sprinkles for a "buttery" taste.

One day before, cut off broccoli stems and thinly slice; cut tops into 1½-inch florets. Cut cauliflower into 1-inch florets. Place cauliflower in center of 2-quart microwave-safe dish; arrange broccoli around cauliflower. Sprinkle with salt, pepper, and water. Cover with plastic wrap; prick holes in plastic wrap with fork; refrigerate overnight. Slice mushrooms in ¼-inch slices, place in covered dish; refrigerate overnight.

On the next day, microwave broccoli and cauliflower on high for 5 minutes. Arrange sliced mushrooms around edge of dish. Cover with plastic wrap and microwave on high for 5 minutes.

Microwave oil in small bowl for 30 seconds; add marjoram and lemon juice; mix. Drizzle sauce over vegetables or serve on the side. Garnish vegetables with lemon slice. Serves 8.

Per Serving:
calories 50
carbohydrate 7 g
protein 3 g
fat 1 g
saturated fat 0 g
cholesterol 0 mg
sodium 90 mg
fiber 5 g
soluble fiber 2 g

Sunshine Carrots

8 medium carrots
1 tablespoon sugar
1 tablespoon cornstarch
¼ teaspoon salt
¼ teaspoon ground ginger
¼ cup orange juice
1 teaspoon canola oil
parsley garnish (optional)

Per Serving:
calories 80
carbohydrate 17 g
protein 1 g
fat 1 g
saturated fat 0 g
cholesterol 0 mg
sodium 120 mg
fiber 3 g
soluble fiber 1 g

Slice carrots crosswise about ½ inch thick. Cook covered in salted boiling water for 15 to 20 minutes until tender. Place in serving dish. Combine sugar, cornstarch, salt, ginger, and orange juice in small saucepan. Cook on low to medium heat until mixture thickens and bubbles. Stir in oil. Pour sauce over carrots and mix gently. Garnish with parsley. Serves 6.

Variations: The carrots and the sauce may be prepared in the microwave.

Pat's "Fried" Corn

4 small ears fresh sweet corn
¼ cup water
¼ medium green pepper, chopped
1 teaspoon sugar (optional)
salt (to taste)
black pepper (to taste)

Per Serving:
calories 80
carbohydrate 18 g
protein 2 g
fat 0 g
saturated fat 0 g
cholesterol 0 mg
sodium 280 mg
fiber 5 g
soluble fiber 2 g

Spray medium skillet with vegetable spray. Cut corn kernels from the cob and place in skillet; make one or two shallow cuts then scrape milk from cob into skillet. Add ¼ cup water and green pepper to skillet. Add sugar, salt, and pepper; stir. Cover and cook over low heat for 5 to 8 minutes until juice is thickened and corn is tender. Serves 4.

Herbed Green Beans

1 9-ounce package frozen
    French-style green beans
⅓ cup green pepper, chopped
¼ cup onion, chopped
1 clove garlic, minced
1 teaspoon olive oil
1 tomato, peeled and chopped
¼ teaspoon salt
¼ teaspoon sugar
¼ teaspoon basil leaves
⅛ teaspoon crushed rosemary
dash black pepper

Per Serving:
calories 55
carbohydrate 10 g
protein 2 g
fat 1 g
saturated fat 0 g
cholesterol 0 mg
sodium 180 mg
fiber 4 g
soluble fiber 1 g

Cook green beans as directed on package and drain. In a 1-quart bowl combine green pepper, onion, garlic, and oil. Microwave on high for 1 to 2 minutes until tender. Add green beans and remaining ingredients; mix and cover. Microwave on high for 1 to 2 minutes until heated. Serves 4.

Summer Mixed Greens

8 cups packed mixed greens, coarsely chopped
   (collard, turnip, mustard, kale, etc.)
2 teaspoons canola oil
½ cup onion, finely chopped
½ cup celery, finely chopped
1 tablespoon cider vinegar
½ teaspoon red pepper flakes
½ teaspoon salt
2 cups water

Per Serving:
calories 50
carbohydrate 7 g
protein 3 g
fat 1 g
saturated fat 0 g
cholesterol 0 mg
sodium 160 mg
fiber 6 g
soluble fiber 2 g

Clean and wash greens; drain thoroughly. Heat oil in slow cooker over medium heat. Add onions and celery and cook for 5 minutes until tender, stirring occasionally. Stir in greens; cover and cook for 10 minutes until greens are wilted, stirring occasionally. Add vinegar, pepper flakes, and salt; cover and cook for 5 minutes. Add 2 cups water, reduce heat, and simmer for 1½ hours, adding more water if necessary. Serve with additional vinegar if desired. Serves 6 to 8.

Variation: Peanut oil may be substituted for the canola oil.

Dilled Fresh Peas

1 cup fresh shelled or frozen peas
2 tablespoons water
1 teaspoon canola oil
⅛ teaspoon dried dill weed

Combine peas and water in microwavable serving dish. Cover and microwave on high for 3 to 3½ minutes until tender; drain. Add oil and dill and stir gently. Serves 2.

Variations: Mix in imitation butter-flavored sprinkles to get that "buttery" taste.

Per Serving:
calories 80
carbohydrate 11 g
protein 4 g
fat 2 g
saturated fat 0 g
cholesterol 0 mg
sodium 70 mg
fiber 5 g
soluble fiber 1 g

Jim's Succotash

1 teaspoon canola oil
½ cup onions, chopped
1 15- to 16-ounce can lima beans, drained
1 15- to 16-ounce can corn kernels, drained
1 cup canned tomatoes, chopped and drained
1 teaspoon oregano
ground black pepper (to taste)

Heat oil in large skillet; add onions and sauté for 3 minutes. Add remaining ingredients; cover and simmer for 10 minutes until flavors are blended. Serves 6.

Variations: Use canned tomatoes with green chilies to make more spicy. To get the traditional buttery, nonspicy flavor, omit oregano, and mix in ½ to 1 teaspoon of butter-flavored sprinkles just before serving.

Drain all your vegetables in a strainer while the onions sauté.

Per Serving:
calories 140
carbohydrate 25 g
protein 5 g
fat 2 g
saturated fat 0 g
cholesterol 0 mg
sodium 430 mg
fiber 8 g
soluble fiber 3 g

Summertime Ratatouille

1 eggplant (about 8 ounces),
  cut into ½ inch cubes
2 garlic cloves, minced
1 small onion, diced
1 small zucchini, thinly sliced
½ medium green pepper,
  cut into thin strips
1 stalk celery, chopped
1 tomato, cut into wedges
dash black pepper
¼ teaspoon salt (optional)
¼ teaspoon basil leaves
¼ teaspoon oregano leaves
⅛ teaspoon thyme leaves

Make ahead;
it ages well.

Per Serving:
calories 60
carbohydrate 14 g
protein 2 g
fat 0 g
saturated fat 0 g
cholesterol 0 mg
sodium 100 mg
fiber 5 g
soluble fiber 1 g

Combine all ingredients into 2-quart casserole and cover. Microwave on high for 7 to 10 minutes until eggplant is translucent, stirring 2 or 3 times. Chill overnight. Serves 4.

Variations: Choose available fresh vegetables; mix in about equal proportions.

Vegetable Strudel

2 teaspoons canola oil, divided
2 medium carrots, cut in strips
1 medium red pepper, cut in strips
1 large onion, chopped
¼ teaspoon black pepper
¼ teaspoon thyme
½ pound mushrooms, sliced
1 16-ounce can red kidney beans,
  rinsed and drained
1 cup (4 ounces) shredded mozzarella cheese
6 sheets phylo dough (12 x 16 inches)
2 tablespoons bread crumbs
paprika

Preheat oven to 375 degrees. Heat 1 teaspoon of oil in 12-inch nonstick skillet over medium to high heat; cook carrots, red pepper, and onion for 3 minutes. Add pepper and thyme; cook for 2 to 3 minutes until tender-crisp. Remove to bowl.

Add 1 teaspoon oil to same skillet over high heat; cook mushrooms until oil is absorbed. Remove to bowl with vegetables. Stir beans and cheese into vegetable mixture.

On work surface spread out 1 sheet of phylo dough; cover with 2 teaspoons bread crumbs. Continue to layer the phylo dough the same way. Spoon vegetable mixture onto dough covering half the dough to within ½-inch from edge. From the vegetable side, roll the phylo dough jelly roll style. Place in jelly roll pan, seam down. Sprinkle with paprika. Cut 12 slashes on top of strudel. Bake strudel for 25 to 30 minutes until golden. Cool in pan 5 minutes. Slice to serve. Makes 6 main dish servings.

Serve topped with one tablespoon of your favorite spaghetti sauce.

Per Serving:
calories 232
carbohydrate 36 g
protein 14 g
fat 8 g
saturated fat 3 g
cholesterol 11 mg
sodium 480 mg
fiber 10 g
soluble fiber 4 g

Marinated Vegetable Medley

1 small head (3 cups) cauliflower, cut into pieces
8 ounces (2 cups) fresh mushrooms, sliced
2 tablespoons water
1 bunch (3 cups) broccoli, cut into pieces
3 green onions, sliced
½ cup fat-free buttermilk dressing
2 tablespoons sunflower seeds
¼ teaspoon water

Per Serving:
calories 80
carbohydrate 13 g
protein 4 g
fat 2 g
saturated fat 0 g
cholesterol 0 mg
sodium 200 mg
fiber 4 g
soluble fiber 2 g

Combine cauliflower, mushrooms, and 2 tablespoons water in 2-quart microwave bowl; cover with plastic wrap. Microwave on high for 2½ to 3 minutes until tender-crisp. Drain and rinse in cold water. Add broccoli, onions, and dressing. Set aside.

Combine sunflower seeds and ¼ teaspoon water in 1-cup microwave container. Microwave on high for 4½ to 5½ minutes until seeds are lightly toasted, stirring 3 or 4 times. Sprinkle seeds over salad.

Cover and refrigerate for at least 12 hours. Mix lightly before serving. Serves 6.

Vegetable Sauté

1 tablespoon canola oil
1 8-ounce package firm tofu, cut into small cubes
1 large onion, cut into thin slices
1 green pepper, cut into thin slices
4 carrots, cut into thin slices
2 stalks celery, cut into thin slices
1 to 2 cups broccoli, cut into pieces
½ medium-sized head cabbage, cut into slices
soy sauce (to taste)
3 cups steamed rice

Per Serving:
calories 210
carbohydrate 36 g
protein 8 g
fat 4 g
saturated fat 0 g
cholesterol 0 mg
sodium 120 mg
fiber 6 g
soluble fiber 2 g

Sauté tofu and vegetables in oil, cover and steam until tender; add soy sauce. Serve over steamed rice. Serves 6.

Variations: Add 1 cup Chinese snow peas and/or 1 red pepper cut into strips. Chicken may be substituted for tofu.

Zucchini Tomato Pie

2 cups zucchini, chopped
1 cup tomatoes, chopped
½ cup onions, chopped
⅓ cup grated Parmesan cheese
1½ cups skim milk
¾ package biscuit baking mix
¼ teaspoon salt
¼ teaspoon black pepper
¾ cup (6 ounces) egg substitute

Heat oven to 400 degrees. Spray 10-inch quiche dish or pie pan with vegetable spray. Sprinkle zucchini, tomatoes, onion, and cheese into dish. Beat remaining ingredients until smooth (15 seconds in blender on high or 1 minute with electric mixer). Pour into dish over vegetables and cheese. Bake for 30 minutes until knife inserted into center comes out clean. Cool for 5 minutes or until firm. Serves 6.

Let it get firm before serving; it gets better the longer it sits.

Per Serving:
calories 150
carbohydrate 20 g
protein 8 g
fat 4 g
saturated fat 1 g
cholesterol 2 mg
sodium 330 mg
fiber 2 g
soluble fiber 1 g

Pizza Potatoes

4 medium potatoes
4 teaspoons butter-flavored sprinkles
¼ teaspoon oregano
¼ cup cooked sliced mushrooms
4 teaspoons chopped ripe olives
½ cup tomato sauce
4 tablespoons shredded low-fat
　　mozzarella cheese

Per Serving:
calories 205
carbohydrate 40 g
protein 5 g
fat 3 g
saturated fat 1 g
cholesterol 5 mg
sodium 220 mg
fiber 5 g
soluble fiber 3 g

Microwave potatoes until tender. Split potatoes and scoop out pulp, leaving shell. Combine pulp with remaining ingredients and spoon into potato shells. Microwave on high 4 minutes or until heated. Serves 4.

Variations: Use your favorite spaghetti sauce instead of oregano and tomato sauce.

Cheesy Whipped Potatoes

6 medium potatoes, peeled and quartered
  (about 2½ pounds)
¼ cup water
3 ounces Neufchâtel cheese
1 cup skim milk
2 teaspoons canola oil
1 teaspoon snipped chives
½ teaspoon salt
¼ teaspoon garlic salt
½ teaspoon butter-flavored sprinkles (to taste)
paprika

May be stored, covered, up to 24 hours in the refrigerator.

Combine potatoes and water in 2-quart microwave casserole. Cover and microwave on high 14 to 16 minutes or until tender, stirring once; drain. Cube cheese and add to potatoes along with skim milk, oil, chives, salts, and butter sprinkles. Beat until fluffy; spread evenly in dish. Microwave, covered, on high 7 to 9 minutes or until heated through, stirring once. Sprinkle with paprika. Serves 8.

Per Serving:
calories 160
carbohydrate 27 g
protein 4 g
fat 4 g
saturated fat 2 g
cholesterol 9 mg
sodium 250 mg
fiber 3 g
soluble fiber 1 g

Colorful Mashed Potatoes

2 pounds small new potatoes, halved
1 pound carrots, cut into 1-inch pieces
1 teaspoon salt
1 tablespoon canola oil
1 teaspoon minced garlic
1 teaspoon ground cumin
1 cup skim milk
1 teaspoon salt
½ teaspoon freshly ground black pepper

Per Serving:
calories 215
carbohydrate 40 g
protein 5 g
fat 3 g
saturated fat 0 g
cholesterol 1 mg
sodium 100 mg
fiber 6
soluble fiber 3 g

Place potatoes and carrots in large saucepan. Add water to cover and 1 teaspoon salt. Bring saucepan to boil over high heat and cook until vegetables are tender, about 15 minutes.

Meanwhile, heat oil in small saucepan over medium heat. Add garlic and cumin; cook 30 seconds. Add milk, increase heat to high and cook until bubbles form around edge of pan.

Drain potatoes and carrots. Return to large saucepan; add hot milk, salt, and pepper. Mash vegetables with potato masher. Serves 6.

Parmesan Oven Fries

½ tablespoon canola oil
1 large baking potato
½ tablespoon grated Parmesan cheese
½ teaspoon chili powder
dash salt

Per Serving:
calories 110
carbohydrate 17 g
protein 2 g
fat 4 g
saturated fat 0 g
cholesterol 1 mg
sodium 90 mg
fiber 2 g
soluble fiber 1 g

Place oil in 8-inch round microwave baking dish. Scrub potato; cut in half lengthwise. Then cut each half into 6 wedges.
Place wedges in dish, coating all sides of potato with oil.
Combine Parmesan cheese, chili powder, and salt; sprinkle
over potato wedges. Cover with paper towel and microwave
on high 6 to 7 minutes or until potatoes are tender, rotating
dish once. Serves 2.

Variations: Substitute cajun or salad seasoning for chili
powder.

SALADS

Apple-Citrus Salad

4 Red Delicious apples, unpeeled, cored,
    and sliced lengthwise
4 medium grapefruit, peeled and sectioned
4 medium oranges, peeled and sectioned
1 cup unsweetened orange juice
¼ cup flaked coconut

Combine first 4 ingredients; cover and chill up to 8 hours.
Sprinkle with coconut just before serving. Serves 12.

Per Serving:
calories 95
carbohydrate 21 g
protein 1 g
fat 1 g
saturated fat 0 g
cholesterol 0 mg
sodium 0 mg
fiber 3 g
soluble fiber 1 g

Carrot-Raisin Salad

2 cups grated carrots
½ cup raisins
¼ cup canned unsweetened crushed pineapple,
    drained
3 tablespoons light slaw dressing

Combine carrots, raisins, and pineapple. Add dressing and
mix. Cover and refrigerate for at least 2 hours. Serves 6.

Tips: We used Marzetti's Light Slaw Dressing.

Variations: You may add slices of celery to this if desired.

Per Serving:
calories 75
carbohydrate 14 g
protein 1 g
fat 2 g
saturated fat 0 g
cholesterol 0 mg
sodium 100 mg
fiber 2 g
soluble fiber 1 g

Anytime Coleslaw

1 teaspoon salt
1 medium head cabbage (about 1½ pounds),
  shredded or chopped
¼ cup water
¼ cup vinegar
¼ cup sugar
¼ teaspoon celery seed
¼ teaspoon dry mustard
dash black pepper
1 medium carrot, shredded
⅓ cup finely chopped green pepper
1 tablespoon finely chopped onion

Per Serving:
calories 60
carbohydrate 14 g
protein 1 g
fat 0 g
saturated fat 0 g
cholesterol 0 mg
sodium 200 mg
fiber 2 g
soluble fiber 0 g

Sprinkle salt over cabbage in large mixing bowl; let stand about 1 hour. Squeeze out liquid.

Combine water, vinegar, sugar, celery seed, mustard, and pepper in 2-cup microwave measure. Microwave, uncovered, on high 1½ to 2 minutes or until mixture boils. Stir; then microwave on high 1 minute longer to blend flavors. Cool.

Add carrot, green pepper, and onion to cabbage. Add cooled dressing; mix well. Pack into 3 freezer containers. Cover, label, and freeze up to 3 months.

To serve, microwave on high one uncovered container at a time 2 to 2½ minutes or until edges are slightly warm. Break up with fork and allow to finish defrosting at room temperature for about 5 minutes. Serves 8.

Fiesta Salad

2 medium sweet red peppers
1 8-ounce can green beans, drained
1 10½-ounce can white beans, drained
1 10½-ounce can kidney beans, drained
1 small red onion, thinly sliced
1 tablespoon olive oil
2 tablespoons lemon juice
¼ teaspoon black pepper
2 tablespoons minced parsley

Per Serving:
calories 125
carbohydrate 21 g
protein 6 g
fat 2 g
saturated fat 0 g
cholesterol 0 mg
sodium 300 mg
fiber 7 g
soluble fiber 2 g

Cut red peppers in half, remove seeds, flatten on a broiling pan. Broil 6 inches below heat for 8 minutes or until charred. Allow peppers to cool, then peel and cut into ½-inch slices. In a large bowl combine green beans, white beans, kidney beans, onions, and red peppers. In a small bowl combine olive oil, lemon juice, black pepper, and parsley. Pour mixture over beans and mix gently. Cover and chill for two hours. Serves 8.

Tips: You could microwave the red peppers until tender and not peel them. However, we find that the time invested in peeling the peppers pays dividends in taste.

Variations: Any type of beans may be used.

Minted Green Bean Salad

¼ cup plain low-fat yogurt
1 tablespoon chopped fresh mint
1½ teaspoons lime juice
1 packet sweetener *or* 1 teaspoon sugar
1 small clove garlic, minced
dash white pepper
1 16-ounce can green beans
    or 2 cups cooked fresh green beans
6 cherry tomatoes, cut into quarters
2 minced scallions (green onions)

In a small bowl combine yogurt, mint, lime juice, sweetener, garlic, and pepper; stir until blended. In a salad bowl combine green beans, tomatoes, scallions, and yogurt mixture. Toss to coat; chill. Serves 2.

Per Serving:
calories 70
carbohydrate 12 g
protein 3 g
fat 1 g
saturated fat 0 g
cholesterol 1 mg
sodium 400 mg
fiber 6 g
soluble fiber 1 g

Lettuce and Orange Salad

2 medium oranges, peeled and sectioned
¼ teaspoon grated orange peel
1 tablespoon orange juice
½ cup plain low-fat yogurt
2 packets sweetener *or* 2 teaspoons sugar
¼ head iceberg lettuce, cut into 4 wedges

Chill orange sections. In a small bowl combine orange peel, orange juice, yogurt, and sweetener; stir together and chill. Place a lettuce wedge on each salad plate and arrange orange sections. Spoon dressing on salads. Serves 4.

Variations: This dressing may be used on a variety of fruits.

Grate orange peel
before peeling
oranges.

Per Serving:
calories 60
carbohydrate 11 g
protein 2 g
fat 1 g
saturated fat 0 g
cholesterol 2 mg
sodium 20 mg
fiber 1 g
soluble fiber 0 g

Mandarin Spinach Salad

6 cups torn fresh spinach (8 ounces)
1 11-ounce can mandarin orange sections, drained
1 cup sliced fresh mushrooms
1 tablespoon lemon juice
1 tablespoon canola oil
1 tablespoon water
½ teaspoon poppy seeds
¼ teaspoon salt
¼ cup toasted slivered almonds (optional)

Per Serving:
calories 60
carbohydrate 9 g
protein 2 g
fat 2 g
saturated fat 0 g
cholesterol 0 mg
sodium 130 mg
fiber 2 g
soluble fiber 1 g

Place torn spinach in a large salad bowl. Add mandarin oranges and mushrooms. Toss lightly; cover and chill. In a screw-top jar combine lemon juice, oil, water, poppy seeds, and salt; cover and shake well; chill. Shake again and pour the dressing over the spinach-orange mixture. Sprinkle toasted almonds on top and serve immediately. Serves 6.

Variations: Use ½ tablespoon oil and 1 tablespoon crushed walnuts with their oil; smash the walnuts further in the oil to make a tasty walnut oil dressing. Crushed walnuts may also be served over the salad.

Company Potato Salad

6 medium potatoes, about 2½ inches in diameter
¼ cup low-calorie Italian dressing
1 cup sliced celery
1 cup thinly sliced red onions
⅓ cup chopped fresh parsley
3 tablespoons white wine vinegar
1 teaspoon salt
dash cayenne pepper

Boil potatoes in skins; peel and slice while hot and place in large bowl. Add Italian dressing. Mix well; chill. Combine remaining ingredients; add to chilled potatoes. Chill until served. Serves 5.

Per Serving:
calories 175
carbohydrate 38 g
protein 4 g
fat 1 g
saturated fat 0 g
cholesterol 1 mg
sodium 450 mg
fiber 5 g
soluble fiber 2 g

Orange-Cucumber Marinated Salad

4 medium oranges, peeled and sectioned
3½ cups cucumbers, peeled and thinly sliced
½ teaspoon orange peel, grated
¼ cup orange juice
¼ cup white wine vinegar
4 packets sweetener or 1½ tablespoons sugar
1 tablespoon minced fresh parsley

Place orange sections and cucumber slices in salad bowl. Add orange peel, orange juice, vinegar, sweetener, and parsley to screw-top jar; cover and shake vigorously. Pour dressing over oranges and cucumbers and mix. Chill for 2 hours and mix again before serving. Serves 6.

Variations: Zucchini may be substituted for cucumber.

Grate orange peel before peeling oranges.

Per Serving:
calories 60
carbohydrate 14 g
protein 1 g
fat 0 g
saturated fat 0 g
cholesterol 0 mg
sodium 6 mg
fiber 2 g
soluble fiber 1 g

Orange Delight

2 cups low-fat small curd cottage cheese
2 cups unsweetened crushed pineapple, drained
2 small packages sugar-free orange-flavored gelatin
2 cups low-calorie prepared whipped topping
sliced fresh strawberries (optional)
fresh mint sprigs (optional)

Mix cottage cheese, pineapple, and dry gelatin; fold in whipped topping. Cover and refrigerate until thoroughly chilled. Spoon into individual serving dishes and garnish each serving with strawberry slices and mint, if desired. Serves 8.

Per Serving:
calories 85
carbohydrate 11 g
protein 8 g
fat 1 g
saturated fat 0 g
cholesterol 3 mg
sodium 260 mg
fiber 1 g
soluble fiber 0 g

Three Bean Salad

1 15- to 16-ounce can wax beans
1 15- to 16-ounce can green beans
1 15- to 16-ounce can kidney beans
½ cup cider vinegar
½ cup onions, minced
½ cup pimientos, chopped
2 tablespoons parsley
2 teaspoons sugar substitute
1 teaspoon salt
1 teaspoon black pepper

Mix together ingredients and refrigerate overnight. Serves 6.

Per Serving:
calories 110
carbohydrate 21 g
protein 6 g
fat 0 g
saturated fat 0 g
cholesterol 0 mg
sodium 380 mg
fiber 9 g
soluble fiber 3 g

Creamy Potato-Vegetable Salad

6 cups cooked potatoes, sliced
½ cup cooked peas, chilled
1 cup broccoli florets
¾ cup thin carrot slices
½ cup celery slices
½ medium onion, sliced or chopped
1 8-ounce bottle buttermilk creamy
    reduced-calorie dressing
⅛ teaspoon black pepper
lettuce leaves

Per Serving:
calories 105
carbohydrate 24 g
protein 2 g
fat 0 g
saturated fat 0 g
cholesterol 0 mg
sodium 310 mg
fiber 3 g
soluble fiber 1 g

Combine potatoes, peas, broccoli, carrots, celery, and onion in a salad bowl; add dressing and mix. Sprinkle with pepper and chill. Serve in salad bowl lined with lettuce leaves. Serves 8.

SOUPS AND SANDWICHES

Healthy Heros

4½ cups thinly sliced fresh mushrooms
3 cups seeded and chopped cucumber
⅓ cup chopped green onions
6 cloves garlic, minced
¾ cup balsamic vinegar
¾ teaspoon freshly ground black pepper
6 2-ounce hoagie buns
12 lettuce leaves
12 ounces thinly sliced lean ham
12 ounces thinly sliced turkey breast
24 slices tomato
1½ cups (6 ounces) shredded part-skim
    mozzarella cheese

Per Serving:
calories 250
carbohydrate 26 g
protein 21 g
fat 7 g
saturated fat 3 g
cholesterol 48 mg
sodium 650 mg
fiber 2 g
soluble fiber 1 g

Combine first 6 ingredients; let stand 30 minutes. Slice buns in half lengthwise; pull out soft insides of top and bottom halves, leaving a shell. (Reserve bread insides for other uses.)

Spoon mushroom mixture evenly into bottom half of each bun; cover mixture with a lettuce leaf. Top lettuce with ham, turkey, tomato slices, and cheese. Top with remaining half of bun; cut in half to serve. Serves 12.

Chive Cheese Sandwich

¼ cup low-fat cottage cheese
2 teaspoons chives
¼ cup (1 ounce) grated Cheddar cheese
¼ cup finely diced celery
8 slices whole-wheat bread

Mix first four ingredients together; serve on bread. Serves 4.

Variations: May be served on English muffins or crackers.

Per Serving:
calories 185
carbohydrate 26 g
protein 9 g
fat 5 g
saturated fat 2 g
cholesterol 8 mg
sodium 460 mg
fiber 3 g
soluble fiber 1 g

Mexican Chicken Sandwich

8 3-ounce chicken breasts, boned and skinned
1 cup prepared salsa
8 hamburger buns
1 cup (4 ounces) shredded low-fat Cheddar cheese
4 ounces avocado, sliced (optional)
2 cups torn lettuce
2 tablespoons chopped green chilies
12 large pitted black olives, sliced

Place chicken breast and salsa in gallon size sealable plastic bag; squeeze to eliminate air and seal bag. Turn to coat chicken. Refrigerate 1 hour, turning bag occasionally. Prepare grill according to manufacturer's directions. Place grill rack 5 inches from coals. Drain chicken and reserve salsa. Grill chicken 8 to 10 minutes, brushing with reserved salsa and turning once. Discard salsa after use. Toast buns on grill, cut sides down, 1 minute; turn and sprinkle the 4 bottom halves with cheese. Grill, cheese side up, 1 to 2 minutes, until cheese melts. Layer avocado, chicken, chilies, lettuce, and olives evenly over cheese; add the tops of rolls. Serves 8.

Per Serving:
calories 370
carbohydrate 28 g
protein 38 g
fat 12 g
saturated fat 3 g
cholesterol 82 mg
sodium 420 mg
fiber 2 g
soluble fiber 1 g

California Club

1 cup thinly sliced unpeeled cucumber
½ cup grated carrot
¼ cup sliced green onions
3 tablespoons fat-free Italian salad dressing
4 tablespoons (2 ounces) light cream cheese
8 slices whole-wheat bread
½ cup alfalfa sprouts

Combine first four ingredients and toss gently; set aside. Spread cheese onto bread. Spoon vegetable mixture over cheese. Garnish with alfalfa sprouts. Serves 4.

Per Serving:
calories 190
carbohydrate 31 g
protein 7 g
fat 4 g
saturated fat 1 g
cholesterol 0 mg
sodium 490 mg
fiber 4 g
soluble fiber 1 g

Veggie Pocket Sandwiches

2 cups chopped fresh spinach
1 cup sliced carrots
1 cup sliced fresh mushrooms
½ medium green or red pepper, chopped
¼ cup fat-free Italian salad dressing
4 4-inch mini whole-wheat pita breads
4 1-ounce slices light Swiss cheese,
    cut into ½-inch strips
1 cup alfalfa sprouts
salt and pepper (to taste)

In large bowl combine spinach, carrots, mushrooms, and green pepper. Add dressing and toss lightly to coat; set aside. With scissors or knife, slit each pita bread halfway around at the seam to form a pocket. Fill each pita pocket with 1 slice cheese, alfalfa sprouts, and one-fourth of the spinach mixture. Season to taste with salt and pepper. Serves 4.

Per Serving:
calories 245
carbohydrate 31 g
protein 14 g
fat 7 g
saturated fat 3 g
cholesterol 20 mg
sodium 600 mg
fiber 3 g
soluble fiber 1 g

Crockpot Black Bean Soup

½ cup thinly sliced carrots
1 small onion, chopped
4 cloves garlic, minced
1 tablespoon canola oil
2 teaspoons ground cumin
2 15-ounce cans black beans,
    rinsed and drained
1 cup fully cooked ham, cubed
¼ cup dry sherry or water
2 bay leaves
1 teaspoon dried oregano, crushed
⅛ teaspoon ground red pepper
¼ cup nonfat sour cream alternative

Per Serving:
calories 330
carbohydrate 44 g
protein 21 g
fat 8 g
saturated fat 1 g
cholesterol 16 mg
sodium 790 mg
fiber 15 g
soluble fiber 6 g

In a 3-quart Dutch oven cook carrot, onion, and garlic in hot oil over medium-low heat for 3 minutes. Add cumin and cook until carrots are tender. Stir in 4 cups water, the beans, ham, sherry, bay leaves, oregano, and ground red pepper. Bring to boil; reduce heat and simmer, uncovered, for 25 minutes. To serve, remove bay leaves and ladle into bowls; top with sour cream. Makes 4 main-dish servings.

Variations: Kidney beans may be substituted for black beans.

Frances' Broccoli Soup

3 15- to 16-ounce cans chicken broth
1 large bunch broccoli (about 1½ pounds),
  broken into pieces
1 large onion, chopped
1 large potato (about ¾ pound), cut up
¼ pound mushrooms
2 teaspoons canola oil (optional)
1 teaspoon curry powder
2 tablespoons lime juice
¼ teaspoon tabasco sauce
sour cream or low-fat yogurt (optional)

Per Serving:
calories 155
carbohydrate 22 g
protein 10 g
fat 3 g
saturated fat 1 g
cholesterol 1 mg
sodium 710 mg
fiber 6 g
soluble fiber 3 g

Combine all ingredients in large cooking pan; cook on medium until vegetables are soft. Set aside ½ cup of cooked vegetable pieces and cut into ¾ inch cubes. Blenderize the rest of the soup, add back the vegetable cubes and serve. Top with a dollop of sour cream or low-fat yogurt. Serves 6.

Tips: The vegetables may be cooked in the microwave, blenderized with the soup and spices, and heated in the microwave.

Variations: Frozen broccoli may be used instead of fresh.

Chili Deluxe

8 ounces ground round beef
1 large onion, chopped
½ green pepper, chopped
3 garlic cloves, minced
2 14½-ounce cans no-salt-added whole tomatoes,
    undrained and chopped
1 8-ounce can no-salt-added tomato sauce
¾ cup water
2 tablespoons chili powder
1 teaspoon ground cumin
¼ teaspoon dried whole oregano
1 16-ounce can kidney beans, drained
1 16-ounce can Mexican chili beans

Heat a large skillet over medium heat; coat with nonstick cooking spray. Add ground round, onion, green pepper, and garlic; cook until beef is browned, stirring to crumble meat; drain. Add tomatoes and next 5 ingredients; stir well. Bring to a boil; reduce heat and simmer, uncovered, 15 minutes, stirring occasionally. Stir in beans and simmer until beans are hot. Makes 6 1-cup servings.

The longer it simmers, the better the flavor.

Per Serving:
calories 300
carbohydrate 38 g
protein 3 g
fat 7 g
saturated fat 3 g
cholesterol 32 mg
sodium 540 mg
fiber 11 g
soluble fiber 4 g

Spanish-Style Gazpacho

2 tablespoons freshly squeezed lemon juice
2 small cloves garlic, minced
2 tablespoons minced fresh dill
    or 1 teaspoon dried dill weed
1 slice day-old bread, crumbled
    (preferably rye or French)
5 large ripe peeled tomatoes
1 green pepper, chopped
4 to 5 scallions or green onions, chopped
1 medium cucumber, chopped
½ teaspoon salt (optional)
coarse black pepper (to taste)
1 teaspoon sugar
1 10½-ounce can chicken broth
tabasco (to taste)

Per Serving:
calories 75
carbohydrate 14 g
protein 3 g
fat 1 g
saturated fat 0 g
cholesterol 0 mg
sodium 210 mg
fiber 3 g
soluble fiber 1 g

Process lemon juice, garlic, dill, and crumbled bread in a blender until smooth. Add remaining ingredients and blend well. Season to taste and chill at least 4 to 5 hours. Serves 6.

Tips: If you don't have an electric blender, use a large mixing bowl, then puree the mixture through a fine sieve. Also, be cautious in using cucumber; too much can overpower the other flavors. Serve in chilled bowls. Pass around bowls of chopped cucumbers, chopped green peppers, minced onions, and croutons for guests to individualize their gazpacho Spanish-style.

Variations: Two 16-ounce cans stewed tomatoes may be substituted for the fresh tomatoes.

Hearty Bean Soup

1 tablespoon canola oil
¼ cup chopped green pepper
½ cup chopped onion
½ cup chopped carrot (1 medium)
1 clove garlic, minced
1 14½-ounce can tomatoes, drained and chopped
2 16-ounce cans navy beans, drained
1 cup water
½ teaspoon salt (optional)
¼ teaspoon black pepper (to taste)
⅛ teaspoon red pepper (to taste)
1 teaspoon sugar
2 teaspoons parsley flakes

Heat oil in a large saucepan; add green pepper, onion, carrot, and garlic and cook about 5 minutes. Add tomatoes, beans, water, salt, peppers, and sugar. Simmer 30 to 60 minutes. Add parsley flakes and cook 5 minutes more. Serves 6.

Per Serving:
calories 185
carbohydrate 30 g
protein 10 g
fat 3 g
saturated fat 0 g
cholesterol 0 mg
sodium 470 mg
fiber 11 g
soluble fiber 3 g

Quick & Easy Vegetable Soup

1 10-ounce package frozen mixed vegetables
1 14½-ounce can beef broth
⅛ teaspoon dried basil leaves
dash black pepper

Combine all ingredients in 1-quart microwave casserole. Cover and microwave on high 10 to 12 minutes or until heated, stirring once. Serves 4.

Per Serving:
calories 50
carbohydrate 9 g
protein 3 g
fat 0 g
saturated fat 0 g
cholesterol 0 mg
sodium 360 mg
fiber 1 g
soluble fiber 0 g

Vegetable Stew

2 teaspoons canola oil
1 cup chopped onion
1 17-ounce can sweet peas (no-salt-added)
1 14½-ounce can stewed tomatoes (no-salt-added)
1 medium red potato, cut into cubes
1 cup chopped green pepper
½ teaspoon salt-free herb and spice seasoning

In skillet, cook onion in oil until tender. Drain peas, reserving liquid. Add reserved liquid, tomatoes, potato, green pepper, and herb and spice seasoning to skillet. Cover and cook over high heat 5 minutes. Uncover and continue cooking 10 minutes or until potato is tender. Reduce heat and add peas; heat through. Serves 6.

Per Serving:
calories 140
carbohydrate 24 g
protein 5 g
fat 2 g
saturated fat 0 g
cholesterol 0 mg
sodium 310 mg
fiber 9 g
soluble fiber 4 g

INDEX

desserts: fruit-sweetened, 30; recommended intake of, 30; suggestions for, 76-77
diabetes, 3, 5-6, 12, 13-14, 37, 42, 51
diet: average American, 5-6, 22-23, 28; balance in, 25-26, 97; for children, 72; guidelines for, 6-7, 11; low-fat, low-cholesterol, 9; 1, 2, 3, 4 food plan, 20-24, 40, 45, 72; in prevention plan, 19-20; and record-keeping, 44-45; vegetarian, 10-11, 30; for weight loss, 13, 36-49; yo-yo syndrome of, 45-46
dietary guidelines, 6-7, 11, 26
Dijon Fish, 160-61
Dijon Flank Steak, 174
Dijon French Bread, 132
Dilled Fresh Peas, 213
dining out. See eating out
dips: Chili Bean Dip, 119; Gingered Fruit Dip, 120; Yogurt Vegetable Dip, 120
diverticular disease of the colon, 15, 16
Domino's Pizza, 103
Down-Home Beans and Beef, 181
drink, tangy tomato, 121
drug use, 58, 63-64
Dunkin' Donuts, 103

Easy Blueberry Crunch, 158
eating, timing of, 33-34
eating out: brown bag lunches, 98-99; from convenience stores, 100; critical skills for, 97; in delis and cafeterias, 101-2; at fast food restaurants, 96, 102-4; at full-service restaurants, 96, 105-10; incidence of, 70, 96; at salad bars, 100-101; and special requests, 97; from vending machines, 96, 100; while traveling, 99-100
eggplant, in Summertime Ratatouille, 214
eggs and egg substitutes, 86
Emily's Applesauce Cake, 158
enchiladas, crowd-pleasing black-bean, 193
Enchilada Stack Up, 192
endurance, 52
equipment, for cooking, 74
exercise: benefits of, 51-53; and blood cholesterol levels, 18, 52; cool-downs after, 56-57; and daily activities, 57-58; and heart disease, 9; plan for, 53-55; in prevention plan, 19-20; safety during, 55-57; warm-ups before, 56, 57; and weight loss, 37, 43-44, 46, 51-52; and wellness, 50-51
eye disease, 14

fast food restaurants, 96, 102-4
Fast Hoppin' John, 184
fats: caloric content of, 27; consumption of, 4, 11, 28; recommended intake of, 22-23, 25-26, 28, 30; shopping suggestions for, 86-87; types of, 27
fiber: benefits of a high-fiber diet, 7-8, 10-11, 14, 19; and cancer, 11-12; and diabetes, 13-14; and heart disease, 8-10; and high blood pressure, 10-11; and hypoglycemia, 15; insoluble, 8; and obesity, 12-13; and other diseases, 15-16; recommended intake of, 7, 23-24; soluble, 4, 8, 32-33; timing of consumption of, 33-34
fiber supplements, 33
Fiesta Salad, 224
fish: caloric content of, 31; preparation of, 31-32, 76; recommended intake of, 28, 31; recommended types of, 31; shopping suggestions for, 87
fish and seafood dishes: Classic Tuna Noodle Casserole, 189; Dijon Fish, 160-61; Jambalaya in a Hurry, 187; Kathy's Seafood Pasta Delight, 188; Marinated Swordfish Steaks, 164; Orange Fish Fillets, 161; Oriental Seafood Stir-fry, 196; Picante Fish, 162; Scallops Supreme, 178; Shrimp Scampi, 179; Steamed Red Snapper, 163; Tomato Flounder, 163; Tropical Shrimp Kebabs, 180
fish oil, 31
five bean dinner, Nancy's, 182-83
flank steak, Dijon, 174
flexibility, 52
flounder, tomato, 163
fluid intake, 34

CPSIA information can be obtained
at www.ICGtesting.com
Printed in the USA
LVOW04*1616160218
566876LV00016B/182/P